# DON'T SNOOZE YOUR DREAMS

## Lessons From Life With Narcolepsy

MICHELLE WEGER

LUCKY BOOK PUBLISHING

"Everything you've ever wanted is on the other side of fear."

~ **George Addair**

# MY GIFT TO YOU

As a special thank you for reading, I'm excited to offer you FREE access to my VIP email list, where I share exclusive surprise bonuses.

You'll receive free coloring sheets as an immediate gift. In Chapter 3, I discuss how taking small steps, like coloring without fear of judgment, can help build the confidence needed to tackle life's bigger challenges.

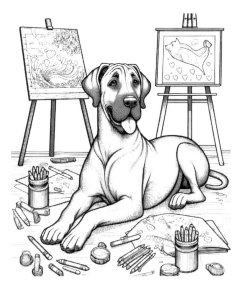

Plus, you'll get a complimentary copy of the "Don't Snooze Your Dreams" Audiobook as soon as it's released!

Scan the QR Code below or visiting

www.michelleweger.com/vip

# PRAISE FOR
# DON'T SNOOZE YOUR DREAMS

*"Michelle Weger's Don't Snooze Your Dreams: Lessons from Life with Narcolepsy is a masterclass in resilience and ambition. With unflinching honesty and a dash of humor, Michelle turns her personal challenges into a roadmap for success. This book isn't just about overcoming adversity; it's about using it as fuel to achieve your wildest dreams. Michelle's story is proof that with the right tactics, there are no limits to what you can accomplish. An inspiring and practical guide for anyone looking to turn their struggles into strengths. I've learned a lot from Michelle's journey, and I know you can too!"*

– **Nick Nanton, 22x Emmy-Award Winning Director/Producer | Wall Street Journal Best-Selling Author**

*"Michelle Weger's Don't Snooze Your Dreams is an incredible roadmap for all of us to overcome our biggest obstacles and live the life of our dreams. She teaches us that life is happening FOR us, not TO us, and every challenge is the training we need to get to*

*our next level. Her DREAM Method perfectly lays out the blueprint for designing an extraordinary life."*

– **Giovanni Marsico, 2x Emmy-Award Winning Producer | Founder/CEO, Archangel**

*"Michelle's book is a powerful testament to the profound impact service animals can have on our lives. As a veterinarian, I've seen firsthand how these incredible animals transform the lives of their handlers, and Michelle's story beautifully illustrates that bond. Her journey with her Great Dane service dog is inspiring and highlights the dedication, resilience, and love that define these partnerships. This book is a must-read for anyone who wants to understand the true value of service animals."*

– **Dr. Sherri Dennett, BSc, Doctor of Veterinary Medicine (DVM)**

*"Michelle's ability to write such a compelling book is nothing short of remarkable. As a producer, I know how challenging that can be. I'm incredibly proud of her for shining a light on her incredible achievements and the vital role of service animals. She's truly the next Jon Katz."*

– **Victoria Boon, Sundance Award-Winning Documentary and Television Producer, who lost the Academy Award to 'March of the Penguins'**

*"Don't Snooze Your Dreams" is not only Michelle Weger's personal journey with narcolepsy, but also a masterclass in how not to sleepwalk through our own lives. Every page of her book reads like a beautifully crafted website - no surprise there! Clear, concise writing, lots of white space around the words to allow the wisdom and the stories to jump off the page and into our hearts and minds. Her descriptions of the "Paper Dragon" and the "Terrorist in Your Head" brought my own fears into perspective. The realization that not all fears need to be conquered is priceless. Michelle is a living testament to what is possible when you refuse to let fear dictate your life. Time to wake up!"*

**– Teri Kingston, TEDx Speaker, Author of 'Get Ready for TED when TED is Ready for You'**

*"Don't Snooze Your Dreams: Lessons from Life with Narcolepsy" is a beautifully inspiring book about persistence, resilience, and the joy of achieving your dreams! The author has a wonderful way of writing that makes it feel as if you're sitting across from her, sipping a latte, as she shares her best tips for pursuing your dreams without excuses. When fear inevitably pops up, as it often does when we're stretching beyond our comfort zone, she has a gift for you there too with smart, practical advice in an easy-to-use framework that you can carry with you for the rest of your life.*

*Her many stories throughout the book give the reader*

*a true bird's-eye view of what it's like to discover and overcome the challenges that accompany a life-altering diagnosis. And even though she and her Great Dane service dogs face some very challenging times, I found myself laughing out loud through much of the book, as Michelle has a fantastic sense of humor to boot!*

*This is a true gem of a book and a great gift for any "big dreamers" in your life!*

> **– Lauren L'Amour, Author, Speaker, Spiritual Life Coach**

*"Oh my goodness, I absolutely adored this book and trust me, you will too! Michelle beautifully transforms her experience with Narcolepsy into a profound guide on life, self-love, and staying true to oneself. Not only does she share her journey for her own growth but also to empower others facing any challenges across mind, body, and spirit.*

*Within this treasure of a book, you'll be treated to a delightful mix of her personal anecdotes, sprinkled with humor and an abundance of compassion. Prepare to dive deep into your own psyche and life as you resonate with her tales. Michelle cleverly incorporates key takeaways and thought-provoking questions after each story to prompt reflections on how various circumstances have impacted you and your responses to life's twists and turns.*

*This book highlighted the power of unity. It's a powerful reminder that our collective strength lies within us all, reassuring us that we're never truly alone in our struggles and that resilience resides in each and every one of us.*

*For those of you who may be searching for that extra push to believe in yourself, to embrace your inner wisdom, and to carve your unique path, "Don't Snooze Your Dreams" is the beacon you've been waiting for, ready to unveil a whole new world of possibilities and inspiration. Let's embark on this transformative journey together!"*

- **Lilly White, Author of '365 Ways to Power Up Your Life', 'Madness, Addiction & Love', 'Into the Heart of Bali'**

*"Michelle's book "Don't snooze your dreams" has given me sensitivity to a condition I was not aware existed before… Her story was captivating, inspiring, touching and filled with much resilience! I loved how she balanced out things with her awesome sense of humor making the reader feel the lightness in her difficulties. For the animal lover that I am, her adorable service dog Max stole my heart, made me laugh out loud and brought me to tears more than once. This book has given me once more a new awareness on how to navigate my own difficulties in areas of my life and has brought me to appreciate greatly my strengths and abilities to go*

*after my own dreams. I am honored to have had the chance to read this book!"*

> **– Ellie Laliberté, Author of 'Letters From You to You'**

*"As someone who suffers from a sleep disorder, Sleep Apnea, this book was indeed a wake-up call - no pun intended. Michelle's story reminds us that life is what we make it. Her determination to pursue her dreams despite the challenges posed by narcolepsy is genuinely motivating. Her perspective has encouraged me to adopt a more proactive approach to my health and ambitions.*

*As a business owner, I was immediately struck by the practicality of the Rule of 15. Michelle's innovative approach to pricing services is not just revolutionary, but also highly applicable.*

*Michelle's story is not just for those with sleep disorders; it is for anyone who has ever faced a challenge and needed a reminder of what is possible."*

> **– Jez John, CEO, Speaker and Trainer**

*"When I met Michelle, she had already been diagnosed with narcolepsy and was on the journey of embracing her discomfort. When we spoke about my work and her narcolepsy, she lit up at the thought that everyone lives with discomfort and uncertainty, but few people*

*embrace it. What so impressed me about Michelle, is that she stopped building systems to manage her discomfort and focused on solving problems for her clients. With this book she's offering a way to help people stop solving for their difference and lean into the strengths you do have to live the fullest life that you can."*

- **Jennifer McClanahan, CEO and Founder of Leverage to Lead LLC**

*"This book is for everyone. Whether you are currently facing difficult challenges or simply juggling life's challenges. The stories and learnings from this book, will help you find a lift to your spirit to soar personal hurdles, and you may laugh aloud a few times--as I did on a few occasions. Michelle's pursuit to be an entrepreneur was anything but linear, and reading her journey and side-journeys, is impressive. She moved forward, laterally, and was anything but stagnant regardless of her hurdles. She has carefully curated a practical set of tools, and shares advice so we can also face our own obstacles and be braver than we thought we could."*

- **Shelley Murdock, Best-selling Author of Healthy & Fit for Life – The Starter Kit for Women Over 50**

# DEDICATION

To Nabil Ould-Brahim, my greatest ally and the smartest person I know, who has always believed in me and supported my wildest dreams.

To my parents, David and Evelyn Weger, for their unwavering love, support, and belief in me. Your encouragement has been the foundation upon which all my dreams are built. Thank you for always being there, every step of the way, and for helping me become the person I am today.

To Melany Goodhue, my best friend, whose unwavering friendship is a constant source of joy and strength in my life. I know we'll be allies for life.

To Taylor Holmes, for your invaluable guidance in advising which stories to include and your help in writing some of the sections. Your contributions were essential in bringing this book to life.

To Becky Bodnar, who first recognized my narcolepsy, leading me to understand and manage my condition.

To Lisa Larter, my incredible business coach, whose persistent encouragement made many of my dreams a reality.

To Maximus, the first and greatest service dog I'll ever have, who taught me the true meaning of unconditional love and bravery.

To Quinn, my current service dog, who brightens every day with her boundless desire to work and cleverness.

And to all my future service dogs, who will continue to support me in managing narcolepsy in the decades to come. Your skills will bring both stability and safety, making every challenge a bit easier to face.

# FOREWORD

**By Lisa Larter**

I remember it like it was yesterday. We had just taken our garbage to the dump and we were driving back home on what we referred to as the dump road. I was around 16 years old at the time, and I was sharing my dreams of traveling the world with my mother when she said it.

She said, *"Lisa, you have to remember you're not like other kids. You have a chronic illness; you can't just go out and do things like this."*

It felt like a defining moment in my young life before I knew what a defining moment really was. I responded back to my mom defiantly, *"I may have a chronic illness but I am not going to let it stop me from doing the things I want to do in my life. If I am sick and I can't at that moment, it's different, but I'm not going to stop dreaming just because I have a disease."*

At the age of 13, after several years of brutal and

invasive testing, many trips to the doctor, multiple stays in the hospital including a week in ICU and two months in the hospital, I was diagnosed with Crohn's disease.

Crohn's disease is a painful and often debilitating illness. When I was a child, I hemorrhaged from my bowel regularly, resulting in my many stays in the hospital and requiring me to be transfused multiple times before they tested blood for things like HIV. My mom was a single parent, and my illness was likely the most stressful part of raising me.

To her, having the audacity to dream big when at times my life seemed so fragile was something she couldn't imagine.

To me, allowing my disease to dictate the vision for my life was absurd. I had big dreams, and they included moving away from the small town I was raised in, traveling the world, one day owning my own business and eventually becoming an author.

I've done all of those things.

John Maxwell said, *"The best excuse is the worst excuse because it's the one you believe."*

I refused to let my autoimmune disease be an

excuse that limited my capacity to dream and live a full life.

We all have excuses for why we don't lean into our dreams and really go for it. Sometimes it's things like time and money, other times it's fear, relationships, or something like narcolepsy.

When I first met and started advising Michelle Weger on her business, I didn't know she had narcolepsy, and I definitely didn't know a lot about what it meant to live with narcolepsy. She presented herself to me as a very ambitious young woman who took action faster than almost any client I have ever advised. After our first strategy session, we mapped out a six-month plan, and she finished everything on the plan within 30 days and came back and asked, *"What's next?"*

I've watched this woman lean into discomfort with humility and grace in pursuit of her dreams. I've witnessed her be discriminated against because she doesn't "look like" she needs a service dog, and yet time and time again, she calmly and politely shows up and advocates for herself and others every single day. I've watched her build a business that now does more than double a month in sales as what she once did in a year. I've seen her show up and give selflessly at events to help others.

I have never once heard her use narcolepsy as an excuse for why she couldn't do something.

*Don't Snooze Your Dreams* isn't about living with narcolepsy.

It's about how to stop living with your best excuse so you can have the life you dream about.

Michelle has accomplished more in her life thus far than 90% of women who run their own business. If she can do this at her age, imagine what is possible for you and your dreams if you do what she shares in this book.

Age can be an excuse too. Don't let it be yours. You still have time. Start today. Start by reading this book.

**Lisa Larter**
*Author of Pilot to Profit,*
*Co-Author of Masterful Marketing*

# PREFACE

If you've picked up this book, chances are you're standing at the edge of your own personal cliff of "What Ifs" and "Maybes," peering into the abyss of potential that lies beyond your fears. You're not alone—I've been there too, staring into that same abyss, wondering whether I had what it took to leap.

I'm Michelle Weger (rhymes with "Eager," which, incidentally, is how I hope you feel about diving into these pages), and I'm here to guide you on a journey that's as much about conquering fears as it is about embracing life's unexpected twists.

Life has a funny way of presenting challenges that catch us off guard and force us to adapt in ways we never imagined. Take my story, for instance. I live with narcolepsy—a condition that means my brain can randomly decide it's lights out at any moment. Yes, it's as inconvenient as it sounds (imagine dozing off mid-activity or, worse, mid-business meeting). But here's the twist: narcolepsy has also been one of my greatest teachers. It's taught me resilience, creativity, and how to face fears head-on, even when those fears are disguised as something else entirely.

This book isn't a sob story about narcolepsy, nor is it a heroic tale of overcoming insurmountable odds. Instead, it's a real, raw, and sometimes funny guide to facing what scares you the most and coming out stronger on the other side.

From falling asleep on a microscope (true story) to navigating the world with a Great Dane service dog who thinks every round of applause is for her (also true), my journey has been anything but ordinary. But here's the thing: it's not about the extraordinary moments. It's about the ordinary ones too—the daily challenges, the small wins, and the times you just keep going, even when it feels impossible.

But enough about me—this book is really about you. It's about that little voice in your head that whispers, "What if I fail?" or "What will they think?"

It's about turning that voice into your cheerleader instead of your critic. It's about finding the humor in the hiccups and the learning in the letdowns.

Through these pages, I'll share not just my story, but also the framework that's helped me turn fear from a formidable foe into a powerful ally. We'll dive into practical strategies, heartwarming anecdotes, and yes, a few facepalm-worthy moments that are part and parcel of the journey.

This book is for those who are ready to stop snoozing on their dreams. Whether you're cautiously dipping a toe into the waters of possibility or you're ready to cannonball right in, this is the place for you.

Are you ready to step beyond fear and into a world of potential?

Are you prepared to laugh in the face of challenges and dance with your doubts?

If your answer is a hesitant "maybe," a resounding "yes," or even an "I'm not sure, but I'm curious," then you're in the right place. Let's explore what lies beyond fear. It's not just about reaching your true potential; it's about enjoying the ride there.

Let's dive in together.

~ Michelle

# MY DREAM

One of my dreams is to speak on 100 stages within 2 years. Can you help?

If you would like me to speak to your audience about not snoozing their dreams, please reach out.

https://michelleweger.com/

# TABLE OF CONTENTS

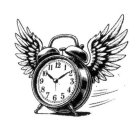

# CHAPTER 1:
# A DREAM INTERRUPTED

## My Journey with Narcolepsy

For most of my life, I wanted to be a doctor. There was a brief period when I also considered aviation. Eventually, I settled on becoming a neurosurgeon with a pilot's license. No big deal.

There was never a question in my mind that this is what I was going to become. I knew I was smart. Most subjects came easily to me in school. I didn't have to work that hard to be successful, but I also wasn't afraid to work hard if I had to. I was enthralled by the idea of medicine: that crossroads of science and compassion. I wanted to be on the forefront of scientific learning, pushing the boundaries of what was possible. And yes, I wanted to heal people. It was a noble pursuit, one I felt was my calling. (And the flying thing—that was just cool.)

I based all of my decisions on this dream: where to go to university, which program to apply to. I really felt I had it all figured out.

My work was rewarded when I was accepted into a prestigious program at Dalhousie University in Halifax, Nova Scotia. Their Diagnostic Cytology (the study of cells to identify disease, such as cancer) program accepts 10 people per year. The pressure was on.

But I was ready for it.

I spent endless hours studying. I glued my eyes to my textbooks. My days and nights blended into a continuous loop of study and lab work. It was tough. But I could see the end goal clearly, so I pushed on.

I was tired, but wasn't everyone? University isn't supposed to be easy.

I still vividly remember the day everything changed.

I was in the lab for an exam. This exam was worth almost half our grade. We would be given three hours to view a series of cells and diagnose them as normal or abnormal. I had studied endlessly for this, and there was a lot riding on it. The professor gave an introduction, turned off the lights, and everyone hunkered down over their microscopes. I put my eyes against the lens, then, in what felt like only moments, I was yanking my head up with an excruciating pain in my eye.

I had fallen asleep, seemingly out of nowhere, on my microscope. My eye was bruised, but it was my ego that took the biggest beating.

*Did I just fall asleep in class?!*

It was in the middle of the school week.

I hadn't been up late.

I hadn't been partying.

There was absolutely no reason for me to fall asleep like that. I'd never done it before.

That first time I fell asleep in public, it was confusing and embarrassing.

The second time was alarming.

The third time was devastating.

Soon I was falling asleep in more classes than I stayed awake in.

How could I ever hack it in this program—nevermind medical school— if I couldn't keep my eyes open?! I was suddenly exhausted all the time. It didn't seem to matter how much sleep I got, either. This wasn't just fatigue; it was a sign of something deeper, something I couldn't just brush off with a strong cup of coffee. My body was dragging me down, and I had no idea what to do.

I went from top of my class to failing. That one failed class alone would be enough to get me kicked out of the program. It was frustrating.

I went to the doctor, and they checked all the normal stuff: thyroid, iron levels, depression. After all, I was 17 years old. Those are the types of things that 17 year olds who are tired typically have. Everything came back normal, again and again.

But I wasn't normal. Something was wrong.

I was still exhausted down to my very bones every single day. In fact, it kept getting worse month after month.

Despite that, I eventually decided to stop trying to figure out the cause and instead figure out a solution. Frankly, I didn't have energy to do both anymore.

Physically, I was barely functioning. Emotionally, I was adrift. All of my dreams, my excruciatingly well-laid plans, were in tatters. I needed to make a change ASAP, before I failed the semester and would have no options left.

---

## Key Takeaways:

- Life's unexpected challenges, like narcolepsy, can derail your plans, but they can also lead to new paths you never imagined.
- Understanding your journey is the first step to overcoming the obstacles in your way.

## Questions:

1. What unexpected challenges have altered your path?
2. How do you respond when life interrupts your plans?

## Fishes of Nova Scotia

When I had to find a new program that I could actually stay awake for, I wasn't looking for something that sparked my interest. I was looking for something that would let me survive.

Enter the Bachelor of Science with a minor in Environmental Science and an area of concentration in Ecology. Although I would come to love these topics, I didn't choose that degree out of passion— it was a completely strategic move.

The degree program had two key advantages:

1. I could transfer all my credits from my original degree.
2. It offered plenty of hands-on field classes.

Instead of sitting in a classroom learning about the Fishes of Nova Scotia (*yes, that was the real name of the course, despite what my editor insists is grammatically correct...*), I would be taking summer classes where I would be outside all day, getting my hands dirty both literally and figuratively. For someone who struggled with staying awake, this was a game changer. Constant movement meant it was easier for me to stay alert, and that meant I could do well despite still being so sleepy every single day.

Of course, there were still plenty of naps, but they happened on the bus rides to tidal pools, mudflats, and frog mating grounds. I took those field classes back to back to back all summer, two summers in a row.

During the regular school year, I chose my classes exclusively based on the time of day. No matter how interesting a class seemed, if it started before noon, it was off the table. Was I riveted by the History of Greece in the 5th Century BC? No. But if it started at 1 p.m., I would seriously consider taking it.

This approach was definitely unconventional, but it worked for me. I was able to do well and complete my degree. In fact, I finished my program in three years instead of the usual four. Despite having switched degree programs because I was failing, I ended up surpassing where I would have been if I had stayed on the traditional path. All because I looked for a way to make things work for *my* situation.

This was the first time I remember actively seeking out ways to do things that worked for me as an individual, rather than following the norm. That mindset has since become a hallmark of how I run my business and lead my life.

At the time, though, it wasn't about being innovative or bold—it was about survival. It was about figuring out how not to end up as a total loser who would be living in her parents' basement forever, which, by the way, was what I kept telling myself would happen if I didn't make this work.

---

**Key Takeaways:**

- Adapting to new circumstances sometimes requires changing your approach entirely.
- Hands-on, experiential learning can be more effective than traditional methods, especially when dealing with physical challenges.

**Questions:**

1. Have you ever had to change your approach to adapt to a new situation? How did it work out?
2. How can you apply experiential learning to your current challenges?

# Camping in the Sudanese Desert

Aside from actually completing my degree, one of the best things to come out of changing my approach to schooling was an unexpected but significant financial benefit: I had money left over.

I had been working part time throughout high school and university to put aside funds to cover rent, food, and other expenses for the duration of my degree. But since I finished a year early, that money was still sitting there, waiting to be used.

I could have done many things with that money.

I could have bought a car.

I could have put a down payment on a house.

Or I could do what every 20 year old dreams of doing: traveling.

And travel I did!

I scoured the internet for trips that piqued my interest and found one that checked off two things I had always wanted to see: the pyramids and giraffes (not necessarily in that order). The trip was a four month-long, rugged, overland journey from Jordan to Kenya. Perfect for someone on a recently graduated, not-yet-working university student budget!

The group of people on the trip was small, and I quickly realized that I was the youngest one by decades. Most of the others were my parents' age or older. I was 20. The next youngest person was 16 years older than me. But age didn't matter—what stood out to me was who these people were.

These were all people who could take three or four months off from work, away from their friends and family, to travel. What that meant, I soon discovered, was that most of them were either established business owners or highly successful corporate employees.

During those long drives through the deserts, we had plenty of time to talk. And if you know me, you know I love to talk. But at 20, I didn't have much to contribute to conversations with people who had decades of life and work experience on me. So between naps, I did a lot of listening. And I learned more than I ever could have imagined.

The corporate types had freedom and flexibility now, at the pinnacle of their careers, but it hadn't always been that way. In fact, most of their careers were spent adhering to the structure of the company culture. One joked that they were glad, as a global VP, to finally have enough clout to refuse 8 a.m. meetings. They didn't begrudge what was required for them to climb the ladder—they thrived in that environment. They took the usual path, and it worked for them. (Boy, did it ever work!)

It scared me, though. I already knew the usual path probably wouldn't work for me - my degree had shown me that. I doubted there were too many corporate environments where I could refuse to show up until 10 a.m. at the earliest. (I might be showing my age here, but this was before the days of work-from-home schedules and a hybrid workforce!)

But then I heard stories from the business owners. They had flexibility far sooner than their corporate counterparts. It came at a cost, of course—they were always "on," always ultimately responsible. But that seemed like a trade-off I could manage.

For the first time in my life, a new idea began to take shape in my mind. Maybe, just maybe, I could start a business. Until then, the thought had never even crossed my mind. I didn't know anyone who had done it, and it seemed like something that only people from movies or rich families could do. But here I was, sitting with real-life examples, role models even, who showed me what was possible.

If I hadn't gone on that trip, if I hadn't met those people, I might never have known that it was possible to start a business without any prior experience. That trip was more than just a chance to see pyramids and giraffes—it was a crash course in what life could look like if I took control of my own destiny. It planted the seed that would eventually grow into my business: Venture Creative Collective.

---

## Key Takeaways:

- Embracing discomfort and unfamiliar environments can lead to personal growth.
- Being the least experienced person in a group can be beneficial if you listen more than you talk.

## Questions:

1. When was the last time you stepped out of your comfort zone, and what did you learn from the experience?
2. What uncomfortable situations have you avoided, and how might facing them help you grow?

# The Accidental Travel Blogger

Before I left for my trip to Africa, I bought an iPad and built a little website. I figured it would be an easy way to post updates and share a few good photos every few days. My family and friends would definitely want to know what I was up to (and if I was still alive), especially since this was before the days of mass social media use. The idea of managing 10 separate email pen pals filled me with dread, and I knew parts of the trip wouldn't even have reliable internet access.

From the first week of my trip, I realized I was going to need help. The internet was often far too slow to upload anything directly to my website. So, I enlisted my mom, Evelyn Weger, to help. I would email her the written content along with a couple of photos, and she would post them to my website using her excellent Canadian internet back at home. Some of the emails took hours to go through, but at least they eventually did if I left the iPad open and connected to hotel Wi-Fi overnight.

Even though my mom had never been on the backend of a website in her life before then, she was eager to learn and help. She didn't care about learning a new skill; she cared about helping her only daughter live her dream.

I felt so fancy—like a travel blogger before travel blogging was even a thing.

*"Your grandma and grandpa love the photos of the ruins!"*
*"Your cousins saw the photos from the mosque!"*
*"Everyone is wondering where you're going next."*

My mom, ever diligent in her new role as part time travel blog editor, replied to each email I sent, sharing who was reading and commenting. One day, she even sent me a little chart from the backend of the website that showed visitor numbers and their locations.

That is how I realized that there were people outside of my close friends and family who were reading my posts. The number of viewers was higher than the number of people I had told about the website. Plus, they were from all over the world, not just Canada where my friends and family were.

This really piqued my interest. Between stops, in places with better Wi-Fi, I started to research how this could be happening.

Turns out, it had to do with something called SEO—Search Engine Optimization. It's how Google decides which websites to show at the top of the search results. I applied what I learned, made a few tweaks to my writing, and sure enough, the views went up again.

This was so cool. It felt like a whole new world was opening up to me. I started proactively reaching out to companies in the towns my tour was visiting, asking if I could write about their day trips or activities in exchange for the cost of the tour being covered..

I admit, I thought it was unlikely anyone would respond to my outreach emails.

But they did! The first yes came within a day! It was a scenic countryside bike trip—an amazing full-day activity. All I had to do, besides enjoy myself, was write about it and take pictures, which I was already doing every day anyway. It was so exciting, and it opened up a whole new world of possibilities—all because I had learned the skill of showing up in searches on the internet.

As my trip continued, my skill set grew, and what was supposed to be just a four-month trip in Africa turned into almost an entire year of traveling around the world. Instead of having to reach out to companies to request to collaborate with them, companies started contacting me to offer me tours.

That year, I got to go to Iceland, Nepal, India, Croatia, Germany, and more. It was an amazing experience, and it all started because I was curious and willing to learn something new. It was also a huge confidence booster.

I never ended up using the Bachelor of Science that I worked so hard for. I didn't need to, because I had found a way to forge my own path.

When I finally decided it was time to come home and start my "real life," I knew I wanted to start a business, but I did not know what kind. With all the confidence of a bulletproof 20-something who had just traveled the world in an entirely unique fashion, I scoffed at the obvious answer: sell the skill set I had built during my travels. Plenty of people wanted nice websites that Google would love, and it would have been a perfect (and reasonable!) opportunity.

But I had just spent months rubbing elbows with people on top of the world (literally—one of the comped trips I took was to Mount Everest!) and was enamored by the thought of doing something more glamorous. (Which is, as I look back, rather ironic since they were the first ones to talk about just how UN-glamorous running a business really is.)

I decided that I would start a super fancy start-up business that an angel investor could one day buy for piles and piles of money.

I knew there was a gap in the market. I knew exactly how to fill said gap. The only teensy weensy problem was that I needed a custom-designed software to execute my idea - the idea that would fill said gap. I knew what components of a website Google loved and how to build those, but I *didn't* know how to build a complex, interactive directory based on location. (The details of this idea don't matter for this story, but if you're curious, send me a DM on Instagram at @daneonaplane and I will send you the original *newspaper* - yes, you read that right - ad for the company.)

I just knew that if I could only get the attention of an angel investor, they would see the potential behind this idea, too.

To practice my pitch, I approached my parents to be my first investors. I remember the initial response from my dad vividly.

He was open, but confused.

*"Why can't you get a normal job like everyone else?"*

Fair.

But my parents saw how hard I had already worked on my shiny new dream, so they offered me a small loan. The money I got from waitressing on evenings and weekends allowed me to pay them back quickly as I worked on my start-up by day.

But despite all that work during the day, I was not making big progress on the start-up business idea. I had all the (perhaps unfounded) confidence in the world, but I had no real framework for facing down my fears and making better decisions. I was even scammed for thousands of dollars (twice!) in the first six months, but that's a story for a future book.

I was settling into life back in Canada. It was at that time that I met one of the people who would change my life.

---

**Key Takeaways:**

- Opportunities come from unexpected places and embracing them can lead to new skills and experiences.
- Being open to learning on the go can lead to significant personal and professional development.

**Questions:**

1. How can you be more open to unexpected opportunities in your life?
2. What new skills have you developed from opportunities you didn't initially plan for?

# The Friend Who Saw What I Couldn't

I credit one of my close friends with my eventual diagnosis. Her name is Rebecca Bodnar, but I call her Becky.

We met at a photoshoot where we were both models. We hit it off immediately, enjoying each other's company throughout the day. At the end of the shoot, I found out Becky didn't have a ride home and couldn't drive. I had just bought my first car and offered to drop her off on my way. That simple gesture sparked a friendship that would change my life.

As people in their early 20s often do, we quickly became inseparable, and that meant plenty of sleepovers. And when I say sleepovers, I really do mean sleep!

We'd plan movie nights, all excited to binge-watch our latest obsessions. But almost as soon as we dimmed the lights and settled in, we were both out cold. Not just nodding off, but dead to the world, absolutely *conked* out kind of asleep. Within minutes.

Both of us. Every single time.

Now, this was completely expected for Becky. She has narcolepsy, something I didn't know much about before meeting her. But for me? I chalked it up to having been chronically exhausted for years by this point. Plus, who doesn't enjoy a good nap during a movie?

But what was just another night for us was actually anything but normal. Ironically, it was Becky who pointed this out to me. She explained that it wasn't "normal" to fall asleep instantly, to be this tired all the time, to lose chunks of my day to these brief blackouts (which are actually called microsleeping - a very brief sleep episode during which you continue to function (talk, put things away, etc.) and then awaken with no memory of the activities). It was normal for her, yes, but she had narcolepsy. What was happening to me was textbook narcolepsy too. Again and again Becky pushed me to get a referral for a sleep study.

At first, I was reluctant. The doctors I'd seen so far hadn't mentioned narcolepsy or a sleep study. Who was I to know more than medical professionals? I figured Becky was just projecting her own experience onto mine.

But Becky wasn't one to back down easily. She made me a deal.

*"If you get a sleep study and you don't end up having narcolepsy, then I will buy all the snacks for all our sleepovers for the rest of our lives."*

Now, let's pause for a moment. All the snacks?! I was only 21. A lifetime of sleepover snacks was a serious offer. And we both knew she couldn't afford it. But she wasn't done.

*"But if you do end up having narcolepsy, then you have to admit forever that I, Rebecca Bodnar, was right, and I am the reason you got diagnosed."*

I mean, what was there to lose? I took the deal and got the referral for a sleep study.

And wouldn't you know it? Becky was right.

That sleep study led to my narcolepsy diagnosis, something I might never have pursued without Becky's insistence. Because of her, I would finally have answers.

---

**Key Takeaways:**

- The support of friends and loved ones can be crucial in helping you recognize and address issues you might not see yourself.
- Sometimes, it takes someone else's perspective to push you towards the help you need.

**Questions:**

1. How can you be more open to the advice and perspectives of those who care about you?

2. Have you ever helped someone else see something they were blind to? How did it impact both of you?

# Testing

A sleep study for diagnosing narcolepsy involves two main parts: the nocturnal polysomnogram (PSG) and the daytime multiple sleep latency test (MSLT). The process is designed to monitor and analyze your sleep patterns in a controlled setting.

I arrived before bedtime. The waiting room was full of older, heavier set men there for suspected sleep apnea. Not too many 20-something, otherwise healthy girls get sleep studies, it turns out. I felt wildly out of place and full of anxiety, which only increased as I saw every other person disappear into a room. I was the last one left in the waiting room.

When I was finally called, I was shown to a private bedroom set up to look like a hotel room. I am sure they do everything they can to make it as comfortable as possible, but there really isn't any way to make cameras and wires look "homey." I felt like I was on a reality TV show. And not the fun kind with wine and roses... It was definitely more "Fear Factor" than "The Bachelor."

The technicians came in to prepare me for the overnight study. They attached sensors to various parts of my body, including my scalp, face, chest, limbs, and fingers. These sensors are connected with wires to equipment that monitors your brain waves, heart rate, breathing, muscle activity, and oxygen levels while you sleep. Although I was able to move and turn, the apparatus certainly wasn't conducive to easy sleeping.

And yet... I fell asleep. Very quickly. As usual.

Throughout the night, the machines and the technician monitored my sleep. The goal of the study is to capture a comprehensive picture of your sleep architecture, including how quickly you fall asleep, sleep stages, any sleep disturbances, and signs of narcolepsy such as sudden loss of muscle tone (cataplexy) or disrupted REM sleep patterns.

The next morning, all those older men got to go home, but I had to stay. The MSLT component of the study measures how quickly you fall asleep in a quiet environment during the day. It's designed to see how fast you enter REM (dreaming) sleep, which is accelerated in people with narcolepsy. You are given opportunities to nap at scheduled intervals throughout the day. Essentially, they put you in a dark, quiet room and tell you to try to fall asleep.

Unsurprisingly, I fell asleep during all five scheduled nap attempts, and even dreamed in each nap. For normal humans, this is highly unusual.

After the naps were done, I was unhooked from all the sensors and sent on my way. Similar to an ultrasound, though, the technicians cannot share any suspected results with you. You have to wait to talk to your doctor.

So I left the study without any answers.

It wasn't until a few days later that I heard from the doctor and found out what had been wrong all along.

---

**Key Takeaways:**

- Diagnosis is a critical step in understanding and managing any condition.
- Testing (medical or otherwise) can be a difficult and emotional process, but it's necessary for progress.

**Questions:**

1. What emotions did you experience during a time when you were being tested or evaluated?
2. How can you support yourself or others through a testing process?

## Diagnosis

Narcolepsy.

The results were definitive and final. There was absolutely no question that I had narcolepsy. I was a textbook case.

I was 22 and had been looking for this answer since I was 17. Five long years. As long as it felt, it was only half the time it takes most people with narcolepsy to be diagnosed. The average person takes 10-15 years to get a diagnosis. Thanks to Becky, my wait was 50% of the norm.

However, this diagnosis came at the most cruelly ironic time.

I had just bought my first car.

It was a brand new Nissan Juke. I had bought it on an eight-year payment plan, which wasn't the smartest financial decision, but I had bought it all on my own and I was so proud of myself. I'd struggled through my degree, traveled the world, and I was making decent money as a server. The car was cute, and it could fit the Great Dane I had just adopted. It felt like a turning point, a symbol of independence.

I even got the very first parking spot right outside

the front doors of my apartment building. Anyone who has experienced a Canadian winter knows how valuable it is to be that much closer in -30 degree weather.

I was driving that new car back from the doctor appointment where the neurologist had given me the diagnosis and told me all about narcolepsy. The car was less than five months old at that point.

Clinically, narcolepsy is a chronic sleep disorder characterized by overwhelming daytime drowsiness and sudden attacks of sleep. It comes with a cast of disruptive companions: sleep paralysis, hallucinations when falling asleep or waking, and disrupted nighttime sleep. It can also include cataplexy, a sudden, uncontrollable muscle weakness or paralysis. Even healthy brains do this in REM sleep to stop you from acting out your dreams. It happens to everyone and is normal. It is to keep you safe. However, in an ironic twist, when it happens during waking hours to a person with narcolepsy, this means falling down unexpectedly.

Wildly, it wasn't until my doctor pointed out instances of this happening to me that I even realized it was cataplexy. Sure, I fell down a lot. I always have bruises. But I thought I was simply clumsy. The extreme tiredness and falling asleep all the time was more obvious, so I didn't really notice the other things happening until I was directly asked about them.

Speaking of that tiredness; they say day-to-day life for a narcoleptic feels like a normal person's experience after 48 hours straight with no sleep. We feel like that all day, every day, forever.

Imagine not sleeping for 48 hours, THEN going to work, driving your kids to school, cooking, cleaning, being nice to your spouse, and socializing with friends. Even after you sleep for a solid eight hours, you will wake up... feeling as if you have not slept for 48 hours straight. There is quite literally no amount of sleep that will ever cure this feeling. I will be forever exhausted.

Within a week I got a letter from the government.

It said in no uncertain terms that I was not allowed to drive. My driver's license was suspended indefinitely. Period. No grace period, no way to appeal. No more driving.

Apparently spontaneously falling asleep was a safety hazard, and the government did not think I was fit to be on the road. And unfortunately for me, they are the definitive authority on the matter.

This beautiful new car I had worked so hard to get immediately became a decoration. Nissan did not accept *"I got narcolepsy"* as a reason to return my car. So the Juke sat in the parking lot day after day, week after week, month after month. That perfect parking spot became torture. Every time I took my dog outside I had to face my expensive, useless car the first moment I walked outside.

I couldn't even sell it.

As is widely known, a new car's value drops the moment you drive it off the lot. That meant that I owed more on my eight-year loan then I could sell the car for. About $10,000 more.

Worse yet, I was still paying full insurance on it!

Medical license suspensions cannot affect your insurance rate in Canada, but canceling your insurance can. I didn't want to be in another expensive situation if I ever did get my driver's license again in the future.

Which, I learned, was unlikely but not impossible. I had found some examples of people with narcolepsy who had eventually earned back the right to drive. I saw them as role models for what could be possible for me long term. But, that was going to be a very long time away, if ever.

Occasionally I would cajole my parents into taking my dog and I for a spin in my car, just so it didn't get rusty. But otherwise, there it sat, a harsh reminder every time I walked out my front door that once again everything in my life had changed.

Despite having wanted answers for so long, I went through a grieving period after getting diagnosed. Even though I was glad to have an answer—finally—about what was wrong with my body, I was grieving the life I thought I would have. I was grieving what *could* have been. I was grieving what should have been. And I was grieving my stupid car.

---

**Key Takeaways:**

- A diagnosis can be both a relief and a challenge, marking the beginning of a new journey of understanding and management.
- Understanding what's holding you back is the first step to overcoming it.

## Questions:

1. How did receiving a diagnosis (medical or otherwise) change your perspective on your situation?

2. How can you use the information from a diagnosis to move forward positively?

## The Way Forward

There was no changing the diagnosis. Narcolepsy is for life. So after I got through the denial phase of my anger, I started to do my research.

I almost wished I hadn't.

The statistics were grim.

**Employment Challenges:** A survey conducted by the Narcolepsy Network found that 38% of people with narcolepsy reported having lost a job due to their condition, and 32% reported being unemployed or unable to work.[1]

**Income Disparities:** A study published in the journal *Sleep* found that people with narcolepsy earn significantly less than the general population, with a median annual income of $25,000 to $34,999.[2]

**Impact on Career Advancement:** According to research published in the *Journal of Clinical Sleep Medicine*, individuals with narcolepsy are less likely to receive promotions or take on leadership roles due to the unpredictable nature of their condition and the stigma associated with it.[3]

**Increased Disability Claims:** A study by the Social Security Administration reported that individuals with narcolepsy have a higher likelihood of receiving disability payments compared to those without the condition, reflecting the significant impact on their ability to work consistently.[4]

**Health Care Costs:** A study in *Sleep Medicine Reviews* estimated that the annual direct medical costs for individuals with narcolepsy are significantly higher than those for the general population, ranging from $5,000 to $14,000 per year, depending on the severity of the condition. This includes costs for medications, doctor visits, and other treatments necessary to manage the condition.[5]

Yikes.

So, if I could even get a job, then it would be for far less money than average, and much of which I could make would need to go to the extra health expenses due to having narcolepsy.

My long abandoned dream of being a neurosurgeon was now laughable. What, would I have to tell the hospital not to schedule any surgeries before 10 a.m., or between 1 p.m. and 3 p.m. so I wouldn't fall asleep hunched over someone's brain with a scalpel in my hand?! Or to make sure that none of the staff made me laugh unexpectedly, or startled me, or else I would collapse on the ground from cataplexy?

No, that occupation was off the table forever now.

And so were most others, apparently. Most day jobs start before 10 a.m. and don't have a napping room, which ruled them out. I didn't relish the thought of telling a potential employer that no, I wasn't lazy, but I couldn't physically wake up before 9 a.m. and that I did actually need to nap every day.

The best chance of success that I saw was to take matters into my own hands. The only way to do that? Entrepreneurship. And not the flashy start-up dream I had been focused on since coming back to Canada: creating the next .com angel investor obsession that I would eventually exit after the business was acquired for zillions of dollars.

That had been a pipe dream. One that I thought was the only way to have a business, because it involved the only type of business owner I had known as role models at that time.

I had been putting in a real effort at creating a startup for the prior 10 months. I spent 10+ hours every day, seven days a week, researching and planning. I had an impressive business plan that was hundreds of pages long. I had lists of potential investors to contact. I was a research and planning machine. And that plan included making money only *after* the start-up was sold.

If it ever sold.

Most start-ups fail.

While I was confident in my idea and tenacity, I also knew I would need a lot of outside help and money, even if things went as well as they possibly could. It was a high risk, high reward scenario that would fail for most people.

While it's not impossible, attaining unicorn status can be incredibly difficult. In fact, a business only has a 0.00006% chance of becoming a unicorn, and it takes an average of seven years for nascent start-ups to grow into unicorns.[6]

Faced with my new reality, that was a risk I could no longer tolerate.

I needed something practical that relied only on my own skills and that could make me money *now*.

I needed to start a boring, local business.

Something that was needed. Something that I could do well, but not something that everyone can do well.

But what?

I thought about a time in my life when I was doing "well," all things considered. Happy, fulfilled, that sort of thing.

My mind wandered off to the days of traveling. Despite the fact that I got lonely by the end of the year, it was a great time in my life. It felt like an easier time. A time when I was managing to have fun, despite being exhausted.

But that wasn't a viable option to go back to.

For one thing, travel blogging was now a saturated market. For another thing, at *some* point I was hoping to have a romantic partner. And I had already learned in my research that only 50% of people with narcolepsy are in relationships, compared to 81% of control groups.7 It was going to be hard enough for me to find a partner, without adding a long-term, full-time nomadic lifestyle into the mix.

*(Now at this point, I am sure you can see what I couldn't at the time. It was probably obvious to you pages ago...)*

DUH!!

It hit me so clearly at that moment; I finally came to the decision that should have been made the year before. But the year before, I was more focused on having a big bold dream. But now? Now I was concerned with creating something that was actually going to work for me in my arguably very unique situation *immediately*. I did not have the luxury of taking years to take a cool idea to market. I needed something to work *now*.

I needed to use the skills I already had - the skills I had built while traveling. Almost every small business needs a nice website that Google loves. And I knew how to do that!

I was going to start a website development company!

Great! That was the plan.

Now what?

I didn't know anyone who had started a small business. The role models I had from Africa were all hugely successful already. I had learned many advanced business lessons from them: the importance of trademarks, clauses to always have in exits agreements, how to value your business for investors, etc. But, I didn't even know the basics of starting an actual money-generating, small local business.

I knew I could not get bogged down in research and planning like I had for the last 10 months. I could not fall back into the trap of endless learning vs action taking; *the more you know, the more you feel like you need to know.*

Those narcolepsy stats were clear; we make less money, work less hours, and stop working younger. Time was truly of the essence.

My mother worked at a hospital, and my father was

in the army. Both had highly structured, respectable jobs. All of my friends were newly out of university, working at traditional jobs. I had no one to ask, "*How the heck do I get started selling something today?*"

So I just... did.

One step at a time.

It's ironic, looking back now. My main motivation for starting a business was fear. I was terrified that my life wouldn't amount to anything. I was terrified to be in poverty. I was terrified to be pitied. So many people are too terrified to start a business, and I was too terrified not to.

But the way I saw it, the risk of not trying was far higher. Worst case, if I tried and failed to start a business, I would be an unemployed person with narcolepsy living in my parents' basement. But that was my current situation.

So my "worst case" couldn't actually get much worse. The outcome would be the same if I tried and failed or if I didn't try at all. But the best case? That could be much, much better. I could become self-sufficient. I could earn enough money to live a comfortable life. I could be fulfilled.

It would be impossible to attain those things without trying.

And every little bit past the worst case scenario, past my current scenario, would make my life better. I would only need a small amount of success to be immediately better off than I was currently. So if I earned a little bit of money, maybe I could get some new clothes. If I earned a little bit more, maybe I could afford an apartment and move out of my parents' basement. A little bit more than that and maybe I could save for a vacation in a few years.

It became a no-brainer. I didn't need to be the most successful; I just needed to be more successful than I currently was.

So, in between a whole lot of naps and taking waitressing shifts at a local restaurant, I signed up for online classes to build on my rudimentary skills in website development and SEO.

Bit by bit, I built a business.

My parents were supportive, but at first they didn't fully grasp what I was doing for work. This was before the days of virtual businesses and Zoom meetings. Few people knew people who had fully virtual jobs. I remember in the early days my dad used to tell people that his daughter *"made money on the Internet."* Which these days means something else entirely! At that point, they were my *only fans*.

But, I was about to find my first client, who would become another supporter.

---

**Key Takeaways:**

- Once you understand the challenges you face, you can start planning your next steps.
- Moving forward often requires a combination of acceptance, strategy, and persistence.

**Questions:**

1. What steps have you taken to move forward after a setback or diagnosis?
2. How do you balance acceptance with the drive to improve your situation?

# My First Client

After doing some practice websites for free or very cheap, it became time to find my first real client. Not an easy thing. I knew nothing about marketing, sales, accounting, or contracts. But I knew how to code and I knew I needed to make my dream of being a self-employed business owner come true. So, I started telling people in my day to day life about my dream. Perhaps one of them would be able to help?

I have noticed that often across the course of my life, when I take the first major step forward towards a big dream, a gift shows up. In my case, that gift was a man named Chris Piper.

Chris is the founder of a project called Man-Kindness, for which he would do random acts of kindness and document them to inspire others. Chris needed a website, and I needed someone who would trust me to make a website knowing I was still new in my business journey.

It was a perfect alignment. I knew Chris because he was a regular at the restaurant where I worked part-time. I had shared with him my dream to take my website development and automation business full time. He wanted to help me. Chris was invested in my dream, because he was invested in me as a person.

That first website was so stressful, but not because of Chris. He was a dream client. But I was so afraid of making mistakes or doing something he wouldn't like. Even though he was the kindest man possible, I was still afraid.

That's normal. What matters is you continue in those scenarios and you don't give up. And you don't let that voice win.

*"You are not good enough."*
*"He won't like what you've made."*
*"This is terrible!"*
*"Why are you even bothering to try?"*

With Chris' encouragement, I kept at it. Because the truth is that nothing is ever perfect, ever. Achieving success happens when you iterate on things over time, ideally in collaboration with others, to create the *best possible outcome*. I worked on that first site for many weeks, and when it was launched, Chris was thrilled with it, and I was too.

Now, comparing it to what we make today, it was rough.

But that didn't matter. If I had let perfectionism take over and stop me from completing the work and delivering it, then the business would have been over before it truly started. There never would have been a second client or a third client, or now 350+ clients.

To this day, over 12 years later, Chris still regularly writes encouraging and supportive comments on my personal and business social media posts.

Talk about a dream first client.

---

## Key Takeaways:

- The beginning of any new venture can be intimidating, but each small success builds confidence and momentum.

- Getting your first client or achieving your first milestone is a crucial step in any journey.

## Questions:

1. How did you feel when you achieved your first significant milestone in a new venture?

2. What lessons did you learn from your first success that you still apply today?

# An Angel in a Dog Costume

Over those early years of growing my website development and automation business, I concurrently dedicated myself to a second very special project. His name was Maximus, and he was a Great Dane.

When I got Max I was in my early 20s, and to be honest, it was a reckless choice. He was being rehomed, and I said "yes" the moment I was offered a dog. I had no idea what I was getting myself into. Of course, I knew that Great Danes are huge (and, for context, I am not. I stand at the impressive height of 5'2). However, I didn't understand what that was going to mean for me. Everything is much harder when your dog weighs more than you do.

When I went to pick Max up, he seemed perfectly sweet. But the moment he was in the car, everything changed. Every person, every car, every trash can we passed turned into a fury of barking. I had never heard a bark like that in my life, and there I was, in a tiny space on wheels, wondering what on earth I had gotten myself into.

But I had made the commitment, and I was determined to follow it through. When we got home, I was thrilled to discover that at least this giant wild animal was potty trained. What he wasn't was leash trained, stranger trained, or anything else trained.

Inside the house, Max was a sweet and loving dog. But the moment he was exposed to something outside of his comfort zone, it was chaos. On our walks, he'd pull me down the street, and I was so embarrassed. Sometimes, I had to use two leashes— one around my waist—so that when he inevitably pulled me and I fell down from how strong he was, at least he couldn't get too far, because he would be dragging my limp body. *I don't recommend that tactic, by the way.*

I kept the curtains closed so he wouldn't see anything scary outside. That kept things calm while we were inside. During those times, I could see the sweet, loving, incredible dog he really was.

Unfortunately, if Max was left alone, such as when I was at work, even with the curtains closed, any noise outside would result in a barrage of barking. For the first six months we were together, I had to pay a neighbor to babysit Max so I could go to work. Half the money I was making was going to dog babysitting.

Yet another reason I hadn't made the smartest decision.

On rare and much-appreciated occasions, a friend

would spend a few hours at my house with Max, saving me that day's dog-sitting dollars. My friend Becky, while babysitting him on one of those days, wrote a poem about Max:

*He wasn't quite a sane Great Dane*
*Not the easiest dog to train.*
*You left him here and it's a crime,*
*Cause he has no concept of time*
*Convinced he'd never see you again*
*The emotionally dependent Great Dane.*

She wasn't wrong.

But, I was stubborn, and Max really loved me. We were in it together.

Over the years, we both learned and grew. I helped him, and he helped me. We worked through his fears of plastic bags, men, and strangers. But when it came to other dogs, there was no chance. I knew by then that his reactivity was rooted in fear, but try convincing other people that your 140-pound dog jumping in the air, snarling and barking, wasn't actually dangerous.

He wasn't just reactive to real dogs either. He'd go nuts over fake dogs, like the seeing-eye dog statues, or even pictures of dogs on walls. He'd even react to the dog on his food bag. I was at a loss. How was I supposed to train this out of him?

I tried everything. Over time, we found some trainers who weren't afraid of big dogs or dogs that did weird things, like freak out at dog food bags. We learned new skills and to adapt. We put the dog food bag in the closet, avoided vet offices with posters of dogs, and only walked him at night. It was a lot of work, but it kept him calm, and he was a great dog—when he wasn't exposed to things that scared him, of course.

Then something unexpected happened. Even before I had been diagnosed with narcolepsy, Max had been doing something extraordinary—at the times I was the most sleepy or doing things that could be dangerous if I fell down, Max would gently put his mouth on my forearm and guide me down to the ground to sit.

Before I was diagnosed, I did not know what he was doing or why. Only after I was diagnosed and Max did the same thing for another person with narcolepsy did it click—Max was alerting for narcolepsy! He knew I was going to fall asleep or fall down before I did!!

How did Max know to do this? My belief is that as a rescue dog Max liked his new home with me and did not want to be kicked out of this new pack. So, he did as dogs do in the wild: he found a job to do for the pack, the family in our case, that no one else was doing. And that job was keeping me safe.

I went on a Google spree. What he was doing was the same as what service dogs do for diabetes and seizures.

This was game-changing. It was the beginning of something remarkable. Imagine having a dog who could prevent you from getting hurt, who could literally keep you safe from yourself. A real life service dog to help me live more easily!

But the reality was, my dog turned into a wild thing when he saw another dog in public. And since there tends to be other dogs in public, there was no way he could ever be a real service dog... Or could he?

My determination to train the reactivity out of him was renewed. We started small, working with him on a higher level of training inside our house and at my parents' house. It started to work. More and more, he was calm around other dogs.

But I wanted more for Max. He was already helping

me so much, and I wanted to help him too. We hired a private service dog trainer who assessed Maximus and guided us through stopping his reactive responses to other dogs.

Max was almost perfect. Almost.

Despite no longer being afraid of *real* dogs, he still reacted strongly to *photos* of dogs.

We were so close! But this final hurdle felt impossible. All the tricks we used to reduce his reactivity to *real* dogs fell flat against the photo nemesis. We were both frustrated.

We needed a change of direction, something to get our mojo back.

So we decided to sign up for some fun trick training classes with a local trainer, Chris Mallick.

In our classes, we learned lots of great things like "chin," "nose touch," and "use your nose." Max loved learning, especially when it was with his family. He would often struggle to do new tricks during the class, but the next day Max would nail them first thing in the morning! Perhaps he had to sleep on them first, which was something that I, of all people, understood.

But there was one trick that seemed to truly stump him. "Use your nose" was about finding a toy or treat hidden behind an object. Max could not grasp this very simple trick.

That is when Chris noticed something crucial—Max never sniffed when he was unsure or afraid! Suddenly, his aversion to dog photos made sense: he couldn't tell that they were not real without using his nose. So in his mind, these *very real* dogs were staring him down, unmoving, which in dog terms is a direct challenge. Real dogs moved, so we were able to teach him that they were not a challenge.

Could it really be that simple to solve this final big issue? Teach Max to sniff on command so he could tell that these stationary challengers were not, in fact, real?

Chris gave us games to play at home that would teach Max to use his nose when asked. We played every day until...

It worked!

I actually cried the first time we passed a dog food aisle without a scene. It had seemed impossible—a fatal flaw in a dog that was otherwise keeping me so safe and making my life easier every day.

This was a journey that took many years. Max was about seven years old by the time he went on his first official outing as a service dog. He retired only a few years later.

Should Max have been a service dog? Well, that's up for debate. His age and history certainly didn't make him a good candidate. But Max really wanted to work. And together as a family we worked so very hard to become a dream working dog team.

What I can say with certainty is this: until you actually diagnose what the *real* issue is, overcoming fear is nearly impossible. The same applies for humans.

Max's story inspired me and many others. A true underdog, my giant reactive Great Dane became a service dog—all because he learned to overcome his fears. And in doing so, Max didn't just change my life; he started a legacy. More on that to come in Chapter 4.

---

**Key Takeaways:**

- Sometimes, the support you need comes from unexpected sources.
- Support systems, whether human or animal, can make a significant difference in managing

challenges.

## Questions:

1. Who or what has been your most unexpected support system, and how have they helped you?

2. Do you have any non-traditional support systems in your life? How can you recognize and appreciate them better?

# The Fear of Being Discovered

In the meantime, on the business side, the fear of my big narcolepsy secret being discovered loomed large over me.

I was terrified that clients—or potential clients—would find out and immediately write me all as less capable, less reliable.

For years I did a perfectly *fine* job hiding my condition… "fine" because I have no doubts that people must have noticed the nodding off, brain fog, and ever present tiredness and assumed there was something wrong with me, but they wouldn't have guessed narcolepsy.

Frankly, the effort was exhausting. Every client meeting, every project deadline was a tightrope walk, balancing my professional persona with the ever-present threat of narcolepsy revealing itself.

This chapter of my life was marked by this constant tension, the fear of my secret being uncovered. It was a fear that shadowed every achievement, every milestone I reached in my business.

And I achieved a lot of milestones in business.

I had plenty of clients and was making enough to sustain myself. (If you recall, that was my entire goal!)

I also met an incredible man, Nabil, who still wanted to marry me even though he knew I had narcolepsy. Imagine that!!

Despite all the wins, I still had this giant secret hanging over me. No one in my work life could find out, because if they did, they'd definitely fire me.

*"Who would want to work with someone like me?"*
*"They wouldn't trust me anymore if they knew."*
*"They would be afraid that I could fall asleep at any time and miss their deadlines."*
*"They will think I am weird."*

The Terrorist in my Head told me many stories about all the horrible things that would happen if people knew my sleepy secret.

I kept my secret for the first four years of business, even when Maximus finished his narcolepsy service dog training.

Despite everything Maximus was doing to protect me, only the people closest to me knew about his role as a service dog. Because only the closest people to me knew I had narcolepsy. There was no way I was going to let anyone in my personal life or business world know my secret.

Until one day, they all found out.

## Key Takeaways:

- The fear of being *"found out"* or not being good enough is common and can be paralyzing.
- Overcoming this fear requires self-compassion and a realistic view of your capabilities.

## Questions:

1. When have you felt the fear of being "discovered" or not measuring up?
2. How can you reframe your thoughts to combat imposter syndrome?
3. What would happen if you let go of the fear of being *"found out"*? How would it change your actions?

## My Dirty Little Secret Exposed

The day I was exposed —like, full-on spotlight-exposed—was in front of a room *full* of people. And not just any people, but some of the most important business connections I had ever hoped to make.

It all started when Nabil and I flew out to British Columbia to visit my grandparents. My entire family was making the trip, too—my parents, my brother, even his baby daughter. It was going to be a full house of family bonding time. But while they were staying a little longer, Nabil and I were flying back a day early. We had a big business event the next day, and we needed time to recharge before diving into all the networking and learning. But mostly, I wanted to fly back a day early because I had a secret to protect.

Maximus had flown with us across the country for the family trip. And while he's more than just a pet—he's my narcolepsy service dog—very few people knew about him.

We were flying into a small local airport, and if we were flying in on event day there was a chance that other event attendees would be arriving at the same time. What if they saw me with Max? What if they figured out my secret? I couldn't risk that. We were flying back a day early to protect me from exposing my secret.

Then, I got an email that threw everything into chaos.

*"I'm looking forward to seeing you tomorrow! Here's some information on parking and other logistics for tomorrow."*

Tomorrow? That wasn't right. Tomorrow is the day we fly home. The event is the day *after* that.

I started to get an anxious bubbly feeling in the pit of my stomach.

I went to double-check the event ticket website before replying back to the host. I was convinced she was going to be embarrassed when I pointed out her mistake. Except... she hadn't gotten it wrong.

The event was the next day. The tickets said so. The website said so. The social media posts from other excited attendees said so.

I had booked our flights for the wrong day.

It turns out I had booked the plane tickets under the influence of narcolepsy. You know those moments of missing memory and microsleeping that my friend Becky pointed out years ago that are a hallmark of narcolepsy? Well, being diagnosed doesn't stop them from happening, especially at night after a long day. I knew the right dates, but

I booked our flights for one day later than I meant to. Instead of arriving a whole day early, we would be landing 15 minutes before the event would be starting.

Fifteen minutes?!

The airport was way more than 15 minutes away from the event venue. But being a little late wasn't my biggest concern. What was I going to do with Max? My family would still be in British Columbia, so they couldn't bring Max home from the airport. So few people even knew about him that I barely had anyone I could ask to help. And of those few, none could take a day off work on such short notice to drive a dog home from the airport.

I started to panic.

This event was a Big Deal. It would be one of the first that Nabil and I were attending together as co-owners of our business. The event was expensive, and I knew it was going to be hugely valuable. More valuable than anything I'd ever spent on a business event before. We had to be there.

I found myself in a lose-lose-lose situation:

If I skipped the event or missed the first half to drive Max home, I'd keep my secret, but we'd miss out on major business connections and learning opportunities. Plus, the investment in the tickets wasn't refundable.

If I brought Max to the event, everyone would know something was wrong with me, and I'd risk losing everything I'd built, just as Nabil was officially joining the business with me.

My husband, being the excellent problem solver that he is, offered to drop me off at the event and then miss it himself to drive Max home. It would have been an easy and selfish "yes" for me, but I couldn't accept his offer. Despite how kind and supportive he was being, I knew he would be disappointed to miss the event. We were a team in both life and business, and this event was supposed to be the first time people saw us as that.

Whatever we chose to do, we would do it together.

I was terrified. The only option left was to bring my service dog to the event. Legally, I knew there were no issues with that. But emotionally? That was a whole other story.

I'd built up so much fear and anxiety in my mind over the past four years. Every horrible worry I'd ever had about revealing my secret came flooding back all at once. But I forced myself to push through it by focusing on how much we'd lose if I threw away the opportunity of this event.

I had made my decision. I was doing it. I was bringing

my narcolepsy service dog to the Big Deal event. I emailed the host to let her know Max was coming. There was no backing out now—canceling last minute would have been embarrassing after asking for accommodation.

It's rare that I say "thank goodness for narcolepsy," but I did that night. Instead of lying awake all night worrying about the next day, I fell asleep immediately, just like every other night.

Good thing, too, because it was an early morning. We boarded our flight before dawn and went straight to the event upon landing. That meant we walked in hand-in-hand, an hour late, with a Great Dane in tow.

I had braced myself for what would happen. Everyone would stare. There would be total silence, followed by a barrage of questions.

*"What's wrong with you?"*
*"Oh, I didn't know we could bring our dogs."*
*"But you don't actually need him, right?"*

Of course, some people would snap photos to share with snarky comments. I was ready for all of it.

But none of that happened.

Sure, everyone looked up (we were late, after all), but no one stared. Not a single negative comment.

The only thing I heard was a quiet "Oh wow, he's beautiful." To which Nabil, with his signature Service Dog Dad charm, responded, *Me? Why thank you!*"

I later found out that the event host, Lisa Larter (who you heard from in the foreword of this book!), had told everyone that we would be late and that we'd have a service dog with us. She'd prepared them for Max's size and explained his purpose. The whole experience was so much easier because of Lisa. She was an ally without me even knowing to ask for one.

To this day, Lisa continues to add a simple line of text to her event info emails whenever we're attending, stating that there will be a service dog in attendance. This removes the shock factor and allows people with allergies to prepare as needed. I still tear up every time I see that line in an email. Her allyship makes it just a little bit easier for us to navigate these situations.

And that's how my dirty little secret got exposed— except, it didn't turn out to be so dirty after all. It was just a part of me, one that I'm learning to be okay with sharing, even if it takes a little help from some amazing allies along the way.

## Key Takeaways:

- Sometimes, the things we try hardest to hide are the very things that make us relatable and human.
- Embracing your vulnerabilities can lead to stronger connections with others.

## Questions:

1. What's something you've been afraid to share with others, and how might sharing it change your relationships?
2. How have your vulnerabilities made you more relatable or approachable?
3. What might happen if you exposed your "dirty little secret" to the world?

# The Repercussions

Nothing could have prepared me for what happened next.

After all my anxiety about bringing Max to the event, after all the sleepless nights I'd had over the years worrying about how people would react to my condition, to my service dog, the first break of the day arrived—and it was nothing like I'd imagined. A few people I knew came over, and then some new faces joined them. They were curious about Max, of course, but more than that, they were kind.

There was no judgment, no awkward questions, no uncomfortable stares. Just genuine curiosity and warmth. It was like this giant weight I'd been carrying around for years just melted away in those first few conversations.

By the afternoon break, something even more unexpected happened. People started pulling me aside for one-on-one conversations. But these weren't just casual chats—they were confessions. These people, some of whom I'd just met that day, began sharing their own secrets with me. They had something different about them too, something they had been hiding. And somehow, seeing me walk in with Max—this giant, furry, "hey, I'm different" sign—made them feel safe enough to share.

The first few times it happened, I didn't know what to do. Why were they telling me this? How was I supposed to react? I was completely caught off guard.

But this wasn't just a one-time thing. It still happens. Every time I go to an event, there's always someone who feels compelled to share their secret with me. Sometimes it even happens in the most unexpected places—at a restaurant, in the grocery store. People seem to feel more comfortable around me because I'm visibly different. My greatest fear had been social rejection for being weird, for not fitting in. But in letting the world know who I actually am, I've somehow become more approachable, especially to those who also have something different about them, too.

That day marked the beginning of a new chapter in my life—one in which I stopped hiding and started embracing who I truly am. And it turns out, authenticity was the key to unlocking so much more than I ever imagined.

My business grew dramatically after that day. We now make more in a month than we used to make in an entire year. And no, it didn't happen just because I brought a dog to a business event. It happened because, with my greatest fear obliterated, I was finally free.

Free from the chains of fear that had held me back for so long. Free to focus on potential instead of playing it safe. When you're operating from a place of fear, you're forced to play small. You're constantly looking over your shoulder, second-guessing yourself, holding back. But once you beat that fear—once you break through that barrier—you become limitless.

I had spent so much energy trying to hide my differences, trying to blend in, trying to be "normal." But that day, I realized something powerful: being different is my strength. It's what makes me stand out, what makes me relatable, what makes me, well, me.

And from that day forward, I stopped hiding. I stopped letting fear dictate my decisions. And as a result, I've been able to achieve more, connect more deeply with others, and live more fully than I ever thought possible.

That was the first day of the rest of my life, and I wouldn't change it for the world.

---

**Key Takeaways:**

- Every action has consequences, and being honest about who you are can have both positive and negative impacts.

- The key is to weigh the repercussions against the benefits of being true to yourself.

**Questions:**

1. What consequences have you faced as a result of being true to yourself?

2. How do you decide when it's worth taking a risk to be authentic

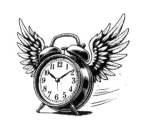

# CHAPTER 2:
# WHAT IS HOLDING YOU BACK

## Impact of Fear on Potential

*We suffer more in imagination than in reality.*

Every time when we're building something up in our mind about how bad or scary it will be, or what other people are gonna think, it's never, ever, ever as bad as you expect it will be.

Never.

Brave doesn't mean not-afraid. It means being afraid and doing it anyway. Over the years I've done a lot of scary things, and I've realized that the ability to do that is the key to getting what you want in life.

The rest of this book is about how I do that. I have created a framework of the steps: DREAM.

Yes, it's a narcolepsy reference. It is also what you

can accomplish if you follow the framework: your dreams! The framework works for everyone, as long as you are going after something you actually really want to achieve.

You have probably noticed by now that I love sharing stories. Each chapter that follows will explain one step of the DREAM framework, followed by a collection of stories. While some are business related, most are not. The stories are not chronologically ordered. My hope is that for each step of your DREAM, you will resonate with at least one of the stories.

The steps of the DREAM method are:

D - Diagnose
R - Role Model
E - Escalate
A - Ally
M - Memorialize

For a more detailed easy reference cheat sheet of the key takeaways of the 5 steps of the DREAM method, go to page 202.

But first, a little science talk (I did tell you I would eventually come to love the science topics I took in university!).

What is fear? Why do we experience it so deeply? And how does knowing that help us?

It all starts with Dinosaurs.

---

**Key Takeaways:**

- Fear has a significant impact on your ability to realize your potential, often leading to missed opportunities.

- Recognizing the ways fear manifests in your life is crucial for taking back control.

**Questions:**

1. How has fear impacted your ability to achieve your goals?

2. What opportunities have you missed out on because of fear?

# The Paper Dinosaur

As different as humans can be from each other, one thing we all share is fear. We all have fears.

This is not a glamorous topic. Most of us try to hide the things we are afraid of.

Napoleon Hill, in his classic book *Think and Grow Rich*, lists the following as the six main fears of humans:

- Fear of Poverty
- Fear of Criticism
- Fear of Ill-health
- Fear of Loss of Love of Someone
- Fear of Old Age
- Fear of Death

Hill's book was first published in 1937, yet this list could be published today and still be accurate. However, I think it's simpler than six types of fears. I think there are two.

To explore this further, let's look at common fears today. When I ask people to list their most common fears, the following often come up:

- Being on live video

- Public speaking
- Skydiving
- Going to an event alone
- Snakes
- Failing
- Water

Is your biggest fear on this list?

Now, let's break them into two groups:

| Type 1 - Physical Fear | Type 2 - Social Fear (aka Brain Trickery) |
|---|---|
| • Skydiving<br>• Snakes<br>• Water | • Being on live video<br>• Public speaking<br>• Going to an event alone<br>• Failing |

Type 1 fears are what I call Physical Fears. These fears all share one thing: you actually could die or get maimed by them. When considering if they are really things you should be afraid of, the answer most times is yes. They could actually have a grave negative impact on your life and that of your family if you choose to expose yourself to them.

Through this book, I will be telling you about the formula called DREAM, which is the way that I use to overcome fears. I do not recommend using the DREAM formula to overcome physical fears. I'm not looking to encourage you to do things that could end up with you injured.

You should not go skydiving with snakes!

The fears I'm hoping you will use this book to overcome are the Type 2 fears: Social Fears. These are every other fear that isn't physical. Although at first these fears seem quite varied, they aren't. They all have one thing in common.

For example, if you're afraid to speak on stage, it's probably because you're afraid you won't be great at it. That would be embarrassing. And then people will think you're not good enough.

Perhaps you'll make a mistake, which could also be embarrassing. And then people will think you're not good enough.

Or maybe you're afraid you'll forget your words, which would be embarrassing. And people would think you're not good enough.

Let's explore another example: asking someone on

a date. If it goes well, you could end up married, or at the very least, with someone you really want to be with. If it goes badly, they could reject you, and you would feel embarrassed. And you would know that they don't think you're good enough.

What's interesting is that almost all non-physical fears are social fears. And there are far more social fears than physical ones in our day-to-day life.

At the end of the day, what we are afraid of is not being good enough. A social fear is not a true fear. It is your brain tricking you into believing that something that is not actually a physical fear is as bad as one.

But why is that? Well, it's something that I call the Paper Dinosaur. Back in caveman times, if we were socially ostracized, it meant being kicked out of the group for not being good enough. That would mean we would no longer have a safe cave to live in or a family to protect us. We would be alone. And at that time, being alone was truly a physical fear.

You would be eaten by a dinosaur or starve, and it would be over for you. You would have no chance to do what we are programmed to do in life, which is to live as long as possible and spread our own DNA as much as possible. Those who respected the social fears got to stay in the cave. Their DNA was spread, and that means most of us came from them.

Back then, the dinosaur was real, an actual physical danger. Nowadays, it's not. What once was a real dinosaur is now a paper dinosaur, an illusion that our brains are still programmed to fear because that's how we survived up until this point in time. But we no longer need to be afraid of the Paper Dinosaur.

You are not in danger of physical harm because you did something embarrassing. A Paper Dinosaur cannot hurt you. Do not fall for the Brain Trickery.

---

**Key Takeaways:**

- The concept of the Paper Dinosaur represents fears that seem larger than life but are actually harmless when examined closely.
- Understanding that these fears are often exaggerated by your mind can help you dismantle them.

**Questions:**

1. What Paper Dinosaurs have you identified in your life?

2. How have these fears affected your decisions and actions?

# The Terrorist in Your Head

As you begin to overcome your fears and beat the paper dinosaur, you will encounter a new enemy. One that is even stronger than the paper dinosaur.

It's called The Terrorist in Your Head. Yes, it's a graphic term, and it's one that I fully stand behind.

The Terrorist in Your Head is the voice that tries to tell you you're not good enough. It's the voice that holds you back and stops you just as you're ready to take those first steps toward a big leap.

*"You aren't smart enough."*
*"People don't like you."*
*"Who are you to think you can do something like this?"*
*"You are going to fail, so why bother trying?"*

This voice has one goal: to stop you from doing risky things, and it perceives going after big dreams as a risk. It wants you to stay safe, and safe means the same. That voice is willing to do anything it needs to in order to achieve its goal, including blowing up anything that is in its way.

The irony is that when you overcome The Terrorist in Your Head for the first time, it won't be over. In fact, it will get worse. The Terrorist in Your Head will get stronger after you beat it the first time, making it harder to beat the second time it comes to visit you.

When you beat The Terrorist in Your Head for the second time, get ready, because it will come back again. And that next time, it will be even harder to overcome.

This pattern will continue onward forever. No one can fully eliminate The Terrorist in Your Head. This is because The Terrorist in Your Head is YOU! That means the stronger you get, the stronger it gets. It is a lifelong game of chess against yourself.

As you work towards making your dreams come true, never forget that voice is there. It will be waiting, ready to sneak back in when you least expect it. It will be there to make you doubt your ability to achieve the things that you dream of doing.

Do not let The Terrorist in Your Head stop you from achieving your dreams.

**Key Takeaways:**

- The Terrorist in Your Head is the internal voice that sabotages your efforts by amplifying fear and self-doubt.

- Learning to recognize and counter this voice is essential for overcoming fear and taking positive action.

**Questions:**

1. How does The Terrorist in Your Head manifest in your life?

2. What impact has The Terrorist in Your Head had on your ability to pursue your goals?

# Conclusion

When it comes to social fears, they often appear one way on the surface but hide a much deeper truth underneath. These fears are the Paper Dinosaurs and The Terrorists in Your Head—those sneaky little monsters that convince us to play small and avoid taking risks. Let's break down a few common social fears and see what they look like on the surface vs what they're really about.

**Fear of Public Speaking**

- **On the Surface:** "I'm afraid I'll mess up, forget what I'm supposed to say, or look foolish in front of everyone."

- **What It Actually Is:** "I'm afraid of being judged and that people will think I'm not good enough, smart enough, or capable enough."

**Fear of Rejection (Asking Someone Out, Proposing an Idea, etc.)**

- **On the Surface:** "What if they say no? What if they don't like me or don't like my idea?"

- **What It Actually Is:** "I'm afraid that their rejection will confirm my own doubts about my worth. If they say no, maybe I'm not lovable, likable, or valuable."

### Fear of Networking or Meeting New People

- **On the Surface:** "I'm worried I won't know what to say, or that I'll come off as awkward or boring."

- **What It Actually Is:** "I'm afraid that I'll be exposed as uninteresting, that I won't fit in, and that others will see I'm not as confident or capable as I want to appear."

### Fear of Sharing Your Work or Ideas (Writing, Art, Business Concepts)

- **On the Surface:** "What if people don't like it? What if they criticize my work?"

- **What It Actually Is:** "I'm scared that if they don't like my work, it means they don't like me. That their criticism isn't just about what I created, but about who I am."

### Fear of Asking for Help

- **On the Surface:** "I don't want to bother anyone or appear weak, needy, or incompetent."

- **What It Actually Is:** "I'm afraid that asking for help will reveal that I'm not as capable as I should be. It's a fear of being exposed as not being enough on my own."

## Fear of Failure

- **On the Surface:** "What if I try and I fail? What if I put in all this effort and it doesn't work out?"

- **What It Actually Is:** "I'm terrified that failure means I'm a failure. That if I don't succeed, it's not just the project or task that fails, but me as a person."

## Fear of Success

- **On the Surface:** "What if I succeed and can't maintain it? What if success changes how others see me, or brings pressures I can't handle?"

- **What It Actually Is:** "I'm afraid that success will expose me. That I'll have to keep proving myself, and that I'll never be able to live up to the new expectations. Success might also mean outgrowing people or places that I'm not ready to leave behind."

These fears are sneaky because they dress up as reasonable concerns, but they're really just the Paper Dinosaurs and the Terrorist in Your Head playing tricks on you. They're trying to protect you from the discomfort of risk, of stepping into the unknown, but in doing so, they're keeping you from reaching your potential.

When you peel back the layers, you see these fears for what they truly are—illusions that are holding you back. They're not real threats, just old stories and beliefs that no longer serve you. The key is to recognize them, call them out for what they are, and then choose to move forward anyway.

The moment you do, those Paper Dinosaurs start to shrink from T-Rexes to Compsognathus (look it up!) and the Terrorist in your head gets a little quieter. It's not that they'll ever fully go away, but once you see them for what they are, you can start living beyond them. You can take that stage, share your ideas, ask for what you need, and know that the real fear isn't in failing—it's in never trying.

---

**Key Takeaways:**

- Identifying and understanding the fears that hold you back is the first step toward overcoming them and reaching your potential.

- By confronting these fears head-on, you can unlock new opportunities and achieve greater success.

**Questions:**

1. What fears have you identified as the biggest obstacles in your life?

2.  How can you start taking steps to confront and overcome these fears?

3.  What opportunities could open up for you if you overcame these fears?

# CHAPTER 3: DIAGNOSE

## What Is Really Holding You Back?

When it comes to tackling the things that hold us back, we often make the mistake of viewing them as one giant, insurmountable wall. It feels like this overwhelming, all-encompassing obstacle that's just too big to deal with. But here's the thing—rarely is it the whole thing that's actually holding you back. Most of the time, it's a few specific parts, and once you identify those parts, the whole becomes a lot less daunting.

The first step of the DREAM method is to diagnose your fear: what is it and what can be done about it.

Think of it like this: You're standing in front of a massive, intimidating structure. From a distance, it looks like one solid, impenetrable block. But when you get closer, you start to see that it's actually made up of smaller pieces. Maybe some of those pieces are loose, or crumbling, or even missing entirely.

And maybe, just maybe, if you focus on those weak spots, you can start to break it down, one piece at a time.

It is like a game of Jenga. The way to win is not to refuse to take out any blocks so as to eliminate the risk of the tower falling over (in fact, doing that will result in no one wanting to play with you again). No, instead you must be aware of the weakest spots, so you don't take blocks out from those spots. You stay in the game by making moves that keep you in the game for as long as possible, so that eventually your opponent will be the one to collapse the tower. Whatever you fear is that opponent, and you can win against it.

This is what diagnosing is all about. It's about getting close enough to really see what's going on, to identify the specific parts that are creating the biggest barriers for you. It's about understanding that you don't have to tackle the entire wall at once. You can start with one brick, one section, one piece, and work on that. Over time, as you chip away at those parts, the whole thing starts to crumble.

But here's the kicker—you have to actually want to overcome it.

Sometimes, when we diagnose what's holding us back, we realize that there are parts we're just not ready to deal with. And that's okay. This isn't about forcing yourself to do something you're not ready for. It's about being honest with yourself about what's truly standing in your way and deciding if and when you want to take it on.

Maybe it's not public speaking that's holding you back; maybe it's the fear of being judged by your peers.

Maybe it's not that you don't have time to start your business; maybe it's the fear of failure that's stopping you from taking that first step.

When you diagnose the real issue, you gain clarity. You can stop fighting against the entire situation and focus on the specific areas that need attention.

And once you've diagnosed the problem, you're in control. You get to decide how to approach it, how to break it down, and how to move forward. You might not solve it overnight, but with each piece you tackle, the whole becomes less intimidating, less overwhelming, and a lot more manageable.

So, let's take a closer look. Let's diagnose what's really holding you back. Because once you see the parts for what they are, you can start to overcome them—one at a time, and on your own terms.

**Key Takeaways:**

- Diagnosing the specific fears and challenges that hold you back is crucial for creating a plan to overcome them.

- Not all fears need to be conquered—some can be acknowledged and set aside if they do not impact your overall potential.

**Questions:**

1. What specific fears or challenges have you diagnosed as holding you back?

2. Which of these fears do you need to address, and which can you set aside?

# A Story About Bubble Baths

I have always been jealous of people who can relax in the bath after a long day. Those bubble bath people seem so happy. They talk about baths like it's as calming as getting a massage, but it can be done in your own home, on your own, any time you want to.

I won't ever be one of those people.

Why?

I could die.

And I swear I am not being dramatic.

They say that it is possible to drown in only an inch of water. A bath is a lot of inches of water. And if you fall asleep in a lot of inches of water, drowning becomes even *more* of a reality.

So, I exclusively shower instead. But even those are something I dislike.

It doesn't help that I have ended up losing up to an hour of time more than once because the warmth and consistency of the sounds from the showerhead lulled me into microsleeping moments.

Perhaps because of this, I don't like water, period. I *can* swim, but not incredibly well, and I certainly don't enjoy it.

So, what's the diagnosis here?

### Diagnosis: Physical Fear... Partially!
### Why?
While it's true that I could actually die if I fall asleep in a peaceful bath or warm shower, it's also true that I'm not going to drift off in a situation with cold water or other sleep-preventing stimuli. So, the fear isn't completely irrational, but it's also not a blanket truth.

### Do I need to overcome it?
Partially! Let's be real—no one wants to be around someone who never showers. So, I do need to manage this fear enough to maintain basic hygiene. But do I need to force myself into becoming a bubble bath enthusiast or a competitive swimmer? Probably not.

### Small Steps:
This fear is a perfect example of why you don't need to go all in at once. There's no need to jump into the deep end—literally or figuratively. It's about taking small, manageable steps that respect where you're at while also pushing you a little outside your comfort zone. So, yes, you will be happy to know

that I do shower, but my showers are cold and short.

**Big Steps:**

One day, I may decide to become someone who swims in deep water. When I'm ready to really tackle this fear, I know who I'm going to call: Stephanie Rainey, the Swimologist. In her adult swimming lessons Stephanie first teaches her students how to stay present and relaxed in any depth of water and second, swim technique—pretty much the opposite of conventional lessons. It's the kind of method that feels right for me, because it acknowledges that fear isn't something you bulldoze through. It's something you work with, piece by piece, until you're ready to take that next step.

So, while I might not be sinking into a bubble-filled bath anytime soon, I'm not ruling out the possibility of becoming more comfortable with water long term.

It's about diagnosing the fear, understanding where it comes from, and deciding how—if at all—you want to address it. And sometimes, it's okay to take the slow and steady route. After all, the goal isn't to eliminate fear completely—it's to learn how to navigate it in a way that works for you, so it doesn't get in the way of your dream coming true.

**Key Takeaways:**

- Some fears are deeply rooted in legitimate concerns, such as safety, and they don't always need to be overcome.

- Understanding when to work around a fear vs when to confront it directly is important for personal growth.

**Questions:**

1. Are there any fears in your life that, like the fear of water, are based on legitimate concerns?

2. How have you chosen to manage these fears— by working around them or confronting them directly?

3. What other strategies can you use to navigate fears that you cannot or do not want to overcome?

# A Story About Coloring Books

If you were to look in my closet, you would see stacks and stacks of coloring books. Under the sea-themed, swear-word-themed, Great Dane-themed. Some just have pages of swirling abstract designs. Beside the coloring books are fancy pencil crayons, fine-tipped markers, and gel pens (yes, the sparkly kind).

See, I decided one day that I needed an extra-curricular activity that could relax me without actively putting me to sleep. As a narcoleptic, most of the usual suspects are out: reading and watching TV are both guaranteed to trick my brain into thinking it is sleepy-time. (I can't count the number of times I have ended up dead asleep only minutes into a show that a friend described as "riveting!") I needed something more active that wasn't actually, well... active.

So I decided on coloring. I am not an artistic person, but I had heard friends talk about how relaxing it is. There is a low barrier to entry. And I could do it sitting down. I was sold!

I went to a local store and bought an ocean-themed adult coloring book and a pack of beautiful artist's pencil crayons. I got home, cracked the book open to a random page, and stared.

And stared.

And stared.

Then, I started to panic. How could I ever decide which colors to start with? What if it looked terrible? What kind of person could screw up a COLORING BOOK?!

I put it away. Maybe the book I chose was just too complicated. Maybe I needed a simpler design.

So, I went back to the store.. This time, I chose a book with an animal theme. The designs were not nearly as intricate. I got home, cracked the book open to a random page, and stared.

And stared.

And stared.

And then I started to panic. The page I had selected had a unicorn on it. Initially, I had grabbed the traditional rainbow colors. (Because rainbows and unicorns seem like an obvious pair!) But then I thought: if the mane is a rainbow, what color should the body be? If I picked a color from the rainbow, that color would be over-represented on the page.

I was filled with dread. This was not fun.

Eventually, I picked a color and started anyway. I picked another color and coloured a different part. I coloured in about quarter of the design before I slammed the book shut in disgust.

It looked horrible. So I put the book away.

I did that more times than I care to admit.

Every time I would start, I would look at what I had done and hate it almost immediately. So I would close the book in horror and get another one. I'd think: oh, clearly I don't have the right color for the skin tone of the mermaid. Oh, clearly I shouldn't have tried to make this dog's eyes hazel. Oh, clearly I selected the wrong green for these leaves...

I was paralyzed.

I was missing out on the mental health benefits of this activity because I was *afraid* that the end result would not live up to arbitrary standards I had set in my mind.

In other words: my fear was impacting my potential.

But, fear of *what*, exactly?

When I thought about it, really thought about it, I realized that the big bad wolf, the fear I was so desperately avoiding, was "failure."

Failure, in this case, meant... an ugly picture.

In a coloring book.

That no one else would *ever* see.

That I could quite literally burn if I wanted to, and no one would know or care.

I was scared that the picture I colored in my adult coloring book would not look *pretty.*

It could not possibly be more of a Paper Dinosaur (well, unless I was coloring a dinosaur on my paper...). There was zero actual danger. Nothing bad could actually happen even if the so-called *worst* scenario occurred: an ugly picture. I was not jumping out of a plane or staring down a venomous snake. When I thought about it that way, it was clear that this was The Terrorist in My Head acting like a toxic jerk, turning this activity that was supposed to be calming and enjoyable into something to avoid and fear.

Digging into the *why* behind the fear exposed my brain for the trickster it was.

I couldn't get more than a quarter of the way through a single page of one of my many, many adult coloring books because I was afraid.

I diagnosed my fear as a fear of failure, which in this case had exactly zero impact on any aspect of my life and was in fact holding me back from accessing the potential mental health benefits of this activity. As a narcoleptic especially, I can't afford to pass up relaxing activities that don't actually put me to sleep within 10 seconds.

I wanted to access those benefits.

Clearly, this was an opportunity I was missing out on. So, I decided to take steps to mitigate the fear that was holding me back. I opted to use a random color palette generator I found online. It would spit out five colors that worked together. I would select those colors from my box of markers and start.

Those were the only colors I was allowed to use, period. No take backs.

Guess what happened?

I had fun! I relaxed. I was able to laugh at some of the pages I created. (The ocean-themed page done entirely in red, orange, yellow, brown, and cream ended up being a surprise favorite!)

Once I got comfortable with "failure"—which, in this case, just meant a hilarious coloring book page I could set on fire if I wanted to—I stopped feeling bad about what I created and finally started to enjoy myself.

That was all I needed. I didn't need to keep progressing, to keep going through additional steps, because I was reaping all the benefits I needed. I had unlocked a relaxing activity that I could reliably use to calm down my brain without falling asleep.

And that was *enough*.

Years later, I still use a random color generator to choose colors for me every time. I don't need to become a coloring guru. I don't need to become an artist.

I am happy with where I am with this. And that makes it the perfect place to stop.

## Diagnosis: Social Fear

### Why?

This was the fear of failure—specifically, the fear of creating something ugly in a coloring book. It is also the fear of being judged, even if the only person judging is yourself. It's the fear that what you create won't live up to some arbitrary standard, and that somehow, that will reflect poorly on you as a person.

### Do I need to overcome it?

Yes, the fear was preventing me from accessing the relaxing, calming effects that coloring could have on my busy brain. As someone who struggles with narcolepsy, finding non-sleep-inducing activities is crucial to my day to day happiness.

### Small Steps:

1. **Remove the Pressure:** I used a random color palette generator to take the decision-making—and the pressure—out of my hands. This allowed me to focus on the activity itself, rather than worrying about making the "right" choices.

2. **Laugh at the Results:** By embracing the possibility of "failure," relax and have fun with the process. Laugh at what doesn't turn out as expected, and move on to the next page.

**Big Steps:**

1. **Accept Where You Are:** I reached a point where I was happy with my coloring skills—or lack thereof. I realized that I didn't need to become an expert or turn this into a serious hobby. I was enjoying it for what it was—a simple, relaxing activity. That was enough for me.

2. **Set Your Own Standards:** I'm good enough at this to be happy, and that's where I'll stay. Sometimes, the biggest step is recognizing when you've reached a place that's just right for you, and then allowing yourself to stop.

By diagnosing my fear, I was able to break it down and take small, manageable steps to overcome it. And in doing so, I unlocked a relaxing activity that I still enjoy to this day. The fear wasn't the whole picture—just a part of it. And once I addressed that part, the rest fell into place.

---

**Key Takeaways:**

- Perfectionism and the fear of failure can turn even simple, enjoyable activities into sources of stress.

- Learning to let go of unrealistic expectations can help you rediscover joy in activities you've avoided out of fear.

## Questions:

1. What activities have you avoided because of perfectionism or fear of failure?

2. How can you start to let go of the need for perfection in these areas?

# A Story About Knives

I don't like cooking.

I'm not good at it, and I have zero desire to become good at it. Why? Because I'm afraid of knives. If I microsleep while chopping vegetables, I could really hurt myself. And I happen to like my fingers... The stress of that fact takes away any potential joy from the activity.

People love to give advice on how to make cooking fun. *"Find a favorite recipe,"* they say. *"Play some music while you cook,"* or *"Prep everything in advance like a cooking show."* Some suggest trying a service like HelloFresh or adding a glass of wine to the mix.

*Spoiler alert*: none of these tips make it fun enough for me to negate the fact that I could cut my finger off.

I know the advice comes from a good place, but it isn't going to change my situation. Can I fry an egg or microwave soup to feed myself? Absolutely. But will I ever cook a meal myself that I cannot wait to eat? Probably not.

The fear at the root of my dislike for cooking is physical, and I'm not interested in working around it. And that is okay!

## Diagnosis: Physical Fear

### Why?

The fear here is grounded in a real, physical concern: the risk of injury from microsleeping while handling knives. This fear isn't irrational; it's a valid protective mechanism.

### Do I need to overcome it?

No. Cooking isn't something I'm passionate about, and this fear isn't holding me back from anything I truly want to do. The risk outweighs the reward, so there's no need to push through it.

### Small Steps:

1. **Outsource:** I can rely on meal services or restaurants, or I can delegate cooking to someone else, allowing me to avoid the risk while still enjoying good food.

2. **Set Boundaries:** I've set clear boundaries— cooking with knives isn't something I'm comfortable with, so I don't do it.

### Big Steps:

1. **Embrace Alternatives:** I've accepted that cooking isn't my thing, and I'm okay with that. I'd rather focus on activities that bring me joy and don't pose a risk.

2. **Own My Choices:** I don't have to justify my

decision to avoid cooking. I'm prioritizing my safety and choosing to spend my energy on what truly matters to me.

In this case, diagnosing my fear helped me realize that not all fears need to be conquered. Some fears are there for a reason, and it's okay to respect them. The important thing is to recognize which fears are holding you back from something you truly want to do and which are simply guiding you away from activities that aren't right for you.

---

**Key Takeaways:**

- Some fears, especially those involving real physical danger, are valid and don't need to be overcome if they don't limit your potential.

- Recognizing and respecting your limits is just as important as pushing past them in areas where it truly matters.

**Questions:**

1. How do you decide whether a fear is worth confronting or simply acknowledging and respecting?

2. What boundaries can you set to ensure that valid fears do not unnecessarily limit your potential?

# Conclusion on Diagnose

Here's the thing: you don't have to do everything.

This book isn't about pushing you to overcome every single fear you have. It's about helping you tackle the fears that are holding you back from things you *genuinely want to do*. It's about determining what you want to do, finding out what's stopping you from doing it, and deciding how to build self-esteem around the things that matter to you.

For example, if there's something you want to try but fear is stopping you, this book is here to help you get through that. But if there's something you don't want to do, and you've identified a valid fear behind it—like my fear of slicing my finger off while cooking—you don't have to work through it. Recognizing and respecting your limits is just as important as overcoming them.

Take bungee jumping, for instance. I'm never going bungee jumping. I have a fear of this activity, and I'm not interested in working through it, because I don't feel limited by not doing it. There are so many people who have gone bungee jumping and rave about their incredible experience.

They tell me, "You're missing out!" And I respond, "The world is a big place. There are plenty of incredible experiences to be had, and I'm not interested in that one."

Why should I work through the fear of skydiving if it doesn't align with my interests or enhance my life? Just because something is amazing for someone else doesn't mean it has to be amazing for you. Embrace your preferences and own your choices.

Bravery isn't about conquering every fear just because—it's about knowing which fears to face and which to accept.

It's your life, and you get to decide what's worth your time, effort, and courage.

---

**Key Takeaways:**

- Diagnosing your fears and challenges allows you to make informed decisions about which ones to confront and which to respect.
- Understanding the root causes of your fears is essential for personal growth and achieving your goals.

**Questions:**

1. What have you learned about the specific fears and challenges that hold you back?
2. How can you use this understanding to make more informed decisions about which fears to address?

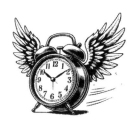

# CHAPTER 4: <u>R</u>OLE MODEL

## Finding Someone Like You

There's something powerful, almost magical, that happens when you see someone "like you" doing something you never thought possible. Until that moment, it's easy to convince yourself that certain dreams are out of reach—reserved for others with more talent, more resources, or more luck.

But the instant you see someone who shares your background, your challenges, or your quirks doing the very thing you've been dreaming of, something clicks.

Suddenly, the impossible seems a little less daunting.

It's like a switch flips in your brain, illuminating a path that was always there but hidden in the shadows of doubt. The obstacles are still there, sure, and they might even seem overwhelming at times. But now, there's a beacon—a shining light that tells you, "If they can do it, so can I."

That's the power of finding your person—your role model. This isn't about idolizing celebrities or chasing after the lives of people you'll never truly know or who are 500 steps ahead of you. It's about finding someone who mirrors your reality in some way. Someone who's faced similar struggles, physically looks like you, comes from the same background or who's walked a path that looks a little bit like yours, and who's managed to achieve something extraordinary despite it all.

Your role model doesn't need to be someone you know personally. In fact, most of the time, they won't be. But that doesn't diminish their impact on your journey. They're proof that the barriers you see aren't as solid as they seem. They're the living, breathing evidence that what you want is possible, even if it still feels nearly impossible.

---

**Key Takeaways:**

- Finding a role model who has overcome similar challenges can provide you with the inspiration and confidence to pursue your own goals.

- Role models show you that what seems impossible is actually achievable, making your own journey feel more attainable.

## Questions:

1. Who are your role models, and how have they influenced your approach to challenges?

2. What qualities do you look for in a role model, and how can you seek out more role models who inspire you?

# A Story About a Guy Who Ran Very Fast

Prior to May 1954, running a mile in under four minutes wasn't just hard—it was considered physically impossible. Until that moment, exactly zero people in the entire history of humanity had ever run that fast.

Everyone, including doctors, scientists, and the athletes themselves believed that the human body simply wasn't capable of such a feat. Physically, it couldn't be done.

Then, in May 1954, something incredible happened! Roger Bannister, a British middle-distance runner, ran a mile in three minutes and 59.4 seconds!

Roger was a good runner. A great runner even. But he wasn't even a full-time professional athlete — he was a medical student! Roger was driven and deeply committed to the belief that he would be the first person to run a sub-four-minute mile, and he made that dream come true!

Roger's accomplishment was impressive. But that is not the reason for sharing this story. What happened next is.

Just one month later, two people ran a mile in under four minutes.

A year after that, five people had done it.

And in 2022, 1755 people ran a sub-four-minute mile. Five of whom were high schoolers!

So what changed?

Did they suddenly start taking some new drugs? Nope.

Did human physiology evolve overnight? No way.

This was a classic example of the power of role models.

The moment Roger Bannister broke that four-minute barrier, something clicked in the brains of others. If he could do it, then so could they. And so they tried to do it too.

As soon as the second person broke the four-minute barrier, it further invigorated the motivation and belief of the others. One person could have been a fluke, a freak of human nature. But, if two people could do it, and so soon, then so could others. And so, they did too.

The four-minute mile had never actually been a real physical barrier; it was a mental one. For years, people had accepted the idea that it couldn't be done, and so they didn't even try. But once people had a role model who showed this was indeed possible, the floodgates opened.

## Key Takeaways:

- The story of Roger Bannister breaking the four-minute mile shows that once someone breaks through a perceived barrier, it becomes possible for others.

- Seeing someone achieve what was thought impossible can be the key to unlocking your own potential.

## Questions:

1. What barriers have you perceived as impossible to overcome, and how has seeing someone else break them influenced you?

2. How can you use the example of others to push through your own perceived limits?

# A Story About Changing Lives

The actions, or the kindness of one person, can often change your life in a significant way. This story is my most impactful example of that.

After some period of working with Lisa Larter as my business coach, the relationship expanded. Lisa owns a company that does marketing, including websites. She started hiring Nabil and me to do white-label (when a company or freelancer does work under the name of another company) website development and automation for some of her clients.

One of those clients was Lisa T. Miller (yes, there are two Lisas in this story). We had the opportunity to build a relationship with Lisa T. Miller over several projects. She is smart, business savvy, and generous. This story starts with that generosity.

In 2019, Lisa Larter was hosting a special event where a small group would go to a bigger conference together (Archangel Summit in Toronto, produced by Giovanni Marsico) and then that small group would mastermind with her the day after the bigger event. It is one of those events that everyone in the room talks about for months afterwards, the kind you're lucky to get into. I really wanted to attend, as did Nabil.

But, we couldn't justify it.

Although our business was doing well, we weren't yet in a place to buy two tickets, plus travel, plus hotel, plus the days off working the business. We would be soon. But not quite then. All costs in, the investment was a little too high for us at that moment.

Lisa T. Miller had bought two tickets to the event but could not attend at the last minute. She asked Lisa Larter if she could gift the tickets to us. We were so excited and grateful! That act of kindness meant we got to attend something that helped our personal and business growth. Something we would have missed out on otherwise.

But for me personally, it did so much more. Being at that specific event changed the course of my life. Lisa T. Miller would likely say that God had a hand in this.

Let me tell you why.

The big moment happened in the auditorium. Lisa Larter had gotten front row tickets for her group. There were about 2,000 people packed into the auditorium, and the lineup of speakers was impressive, to say the least.

Seth Godin was one of the headliners, and he was everything you'd expect—brilliant, insightful, engaging. But it wasn't Seth who flipped the switch in my brain that day. It was another speaker, a woman named Haben Girma, who completely altered what I thought could be possible in my professional life.

Haben is a deaf-blind graduate of Harvard School of Law. She's incredibly smart and very funny. But none of that was what impacted me the most. What struck me—what truly shifted something deep inside me—was that she had a service dog on stage with her.

Now, you have to understand, I had this ingrained belief that you just couldn't do that. You can't bring a service dog on stage.

*What if the dog gets bored?*
*What if he has to pee?*
*What if someone in the audience is afraid of dogs?*

These were the stories The Terrorist in My Head had been telling myself about a service dog being on stage—the same stories that had kept me from bringing my own service dog, Max, to the very event I was sitting in that day.

As I watched Haben stand there, confident and composed, on a massive prestigious stage with her service dog by her side, those stories shattered. In an instant, what I had thought was impossible became possible. My switch was flipped. All those excuses, all those fears I'd clung to, dissolved.

I sat there in the front row, tears streaming down my face, because the truth was, I hadn't brought Max with me to the event because I didn't want to bother anyone. Everyone I knew there already knew about my service dog. They had all asked me why I did not bring him. I sheepishly admitted that I had put worries of others' potential discomfort over my own rights and needs. And because of that, I'd been struggling all morning. I was falling asleep during each speaker, missing those powerful, impactful moments that I was there to absorb. I was angry with myself, upset that I had limited my own potential because of fear of the *potential* discomfort of others. A total Paper Dinosaur.

That day, I made a promise to myself: I would never, ever leave my service dog at home again. After the event, I had the incredible honor of speaking with Haben. I told her what I had done and that it wouldn't happen again. I wanted her to know the impact she had on me. Often, we do not take the time to share our appreciation with the people we see as Role Models.

Haben was the first, and still only, speaker with a service dog that I have seen on a stage... other than myself! In 2023 I started being asked to speak on stages and do TV appearances. I had not been seeking out the opportunities; people were reaching out to me! So, I said, "Yes."

I learned long ago that when several doors open on the same topic in a short period of time, there is a reason. You are meant to go through them. Something life changing is waiting for you on the other side. If you are brave enough to take the steps forward.

So, I did.

Very quickly, people started coming up to me to share the impact I had on them.

I never planned to be a speaker. I did not even think that people with service dogs would get hired to speak at big events before I saw Haben. But when these doors started to open for me, I knew it was indeed possible, because I had seen Haben do it.

I knew this was my opportunity to be a role model for others.

If Haben could stand up there with her service dog and change lives, then I could do it too. And I've been doing it ever since. Each stage I step onto, I do it with my service dog by my side, a living testament to what's possible when you refuse to let fear dictate your life.

If she could do it, then so could I! So now, so can

you (shatter glass ceilings, not specifically the stage-with-a-service-dog thing, that would be weird!)

You will do incredible things of your own. I know it.

---

**Key Takeaways:**

- You have the potential to take an action or give a gift that could change someone else's life.

- Seeing someone like you achieve great things can flip a switch in your mind, turning the impossible into the possible.

**Questions:**

1. What gift could you give to someone that could change their life?

2. What moment in your life made you realize that something you thought was impossible was actually within reach?

# A Story About Training Service Dogs

In 2021 my friend Dr Wendy Rice pulled me aside and gently told me that I needed to plan for a replacement service dog. I didn't want to hear it, and she knew that. But she told me anyway, because she knew how important it was for me to have a service dog to stop me from falling down and falling asleep in public.

Wendy was right, of course. As much as I wanted to pretend that Max would live forever, I knew that was delusional. If I did not plan for what would inevitably happen, then I would be in a bad spot in a few years.

So, the planning began. I started to search for Narcolepsy Service Dog charities. There were none. Then Narcolepsy Service Dog training schools. None. Even searches for private trainers who specialized in Narcolepsy Service Dog came up empty.

This was not going to be easy.

Since Max started alerting to narcolepsy without being trained to do it, we did not know how to actually *train* that skill. I tried to find how others had done it. Narcolepsy is so rare that I had trouble finding more than a handful of other narcoleptics with service dogs out there. The few I could find all had a similar story: their dog started to alert on its own, then they went into professional service dog training. How familiar!

As I pondered how I could find a protege for Maximus, I noticed an interesting example of Role Models happening around me. Many of my friends were having their second child. In every instance, the younger child was hitting developmental milestones faster than the first had. They were watching their older siblings and copying them. But, why didn't the same happen for the first child who had parents they could see and copy?

It was a classic Role Model example: while the adults around them were examples of what human bodies can do (crawl, walk, talk, etc.), it was their older siblings who were closer to their age and size. In order to keep up with them, the younger children would copy the more accessible example of what was possible for them. Thus, the second children were reaching developmental milestones sooner despite, arguably, getting less one-on-one time from their parents.

Could the same be true for dogs?

I managed to find some secondhand accounts of

service dogs in training learning faster when they were trained alongside a fully trained service dog. No one I found had done it themselves though.

So we took the bet that, on top of all the other great things that Max could do, he could also be a great teacher.

What could go wrong? ...Right?

Nothing, as it turns out! The unfounded plan, based solely on a handful of "I know someone who knows someone who did it this way" stories and my deep belief in the power of role models, rolled out like a dream.

We applied for the waitlist to get a Great Dane puppy from one of the best breeders of Champion show dog Great Danes. We had to fly across the country to get her, but it was worth the time and cost. If we were going to gamble that a dog could train a dog, then we wanted to be sure that they came from ethically bred, health tested, proven, sound parents and grandparents.

**I do not recommend a Great Dane as a service dog.** In fact, I do not recommend Great Danes in general for most families. They are truly a great expense; everything costs more for a giant dog. For example, my current Great Dane eats $30 per day in food. Yes, per day. Please do not let these sweet stories lead you to believe that there is anything easy about having a giant dog. It is truly a giant commitment.

The little puppy was already 24lbs the day we flew back home. It was also a Great Dane, like Max, and even the same color. The only difference was that she is a girl. We had hoped for a boy, to try our best for the new prospect to see every part of themselves in Max, but the best service dog prospect in the litter was a girl. So a girl we got!

Her registered name is Paquestone's Quinn Essential, but we call her Quinn. I loved her the moment I met her. Max, however, did not.

Long gone were the days of Max reacting to other dogs, real or fake, negatively. He had become dog neutral years ago. It is a great trait in a service dog, but not the most welcoming to a new puppy. Max was never mean, but he did not go out of his way to love Quinn either. It turns out, that was part of what worked so well for the training.

As a typical puppy (and little sister), Quinn was obsessed with her new older brother. Not only did she follow him around the house all day, she copied everything he did. If Quinn was not sleeping, she was by Max's side, trying so hard to impress him.

Max clearly knew this. He acted indifferent to Quinn most of the time, except for when Quinn did something good. In those moments he would give her a little lick on her head or back. Sometimes, when Quinn was particularly great, Max would let her cuddle with him. Quinn basked in the joy of that approval. She thrived on it and wanted more and more.

For the first three months of Quinn being with us, we would take both her and Max out to work. Max would wear his service dog vest and Quinn would have a badge that said, "In training." Her leash was tied to Max's vest to keep her beside him, so she could easily match his speed and pace to make it easier to copy him.

It worked so well. Everything was three times easier

to train for than we had experienced with Max. Of course it was! Quinn had an example of someone just like her to show her exactly what to do in every situation. She soon earned her own vest and was no longer tied to Max while working.

Don't get me wrong, we still had to do a tremendous amount of training, including many group dog classes, dog sports, and private professional work. Even with a role model, this was a many tens of thousands of dollars endeavor. What was easier was the pace at which the training happened and the enjoyment of the experience.

Despite how well the initial training was going, even we were surprised when, at only four months old, Quinn alerted for narcolepsy for the first time. That had been the biggest gamble, the biggest "what if": what if she couldn't learn that particular skill from Max?

Now, to be fair, she also tackled me to the ground instead of gently guiding me as Max always had. But she learned on the spot from a stern look Max gave her that *"we don't do it like that."*

Sure enough, the next time was much more gentle. As was every time after that. Every lesson was faster and easier, because she had a role model with her

24/7 showing her *"this is what good Great Dane service dogs do for narcoleptics."*

The last day that Max worked in public was my birthday that year. Max was 11 years old and Quinn was five months old. Quinn was almost as big as Max by then. We were in Toronto for a dog show, where Nabil and Quinn ran in circles for a man in a suit (more on that in Chapter 7). After show time, we made the most of our time away from home. We went to the aquarium and then to the CN Tower's spinning restaurant in the sky for dinner.

My favorite part of the beautiful day was at the end of the dinner, when we stood up from our seats to leave and there were audible gasps of surprise when two Great Danes came out from under our table. No one who hadn't seen us arrive hours ago knew either of them were there. It was like a magic show.

Presto, Great Dane! Ta-da!

It was a long, full, day. It felt to me like a crash course service dog test:

- Being around hundreds of other dogs
- A loud place filled with kids
- Riding up 117 stories in an elevator

- Stingrays in open pools
- Riding a conveyor belt through a tank full of sharks
- A long, multicourse dinner in the sky

Max must have felt the same way too. The next time we told them to get their vests to "go working," only Quinn did. Max stayed on the couch, wagging his tail and making it clear that he was happy to stay right where he was.

Max had retired.

Quinn didn't miss a beat and thrived in her new role as a solo service dog. You could tell she was proud of herself, and that Max was too. From that day until the day that he died, Max never again refused to cuddle with Quinn. She had earned his love by taking on the role that Max had always considered to be the most important thing in his world: making sure I was safe.

---

**Key Takeaways:**

- The journey of training a service dog reflects that the power of a role model spans past the human realm.
- Even the most unlikely candidates can rise to

the occasion in their own lives to become a role model to others.

## Questions:

1. How have you or someone you know risen to the occasion despite initial doubts or obstacles?

2. How can you apply the lessons from training a service dog to your own personal or professional growth?

# Conclusion on Role Model

How do you find this person for yourself? How do you identify the role model who can help light the way on your individual journey?

It starts with looking beyond the obvious. Your role model is most likely not in your immediate circle, and they most likely are not super famous (yet, at least!). They might be someone who's quietly making strides in their field, someone whose story isn't widely known but resonates with your own. It might take some digging, some research, and a willingness to step outside your comfort zone to find them. But find them you must.

Because once you do, everything changes. That person becomes the example you can look to when the doubts creep in, when the fear tells you to give up. They become the voice in your head that counters the negativity, that whispers, *"Yes, you can."*

**Ways to Find Role Models:**

1. **Books and Biographies:**

   - Dive into the lives of inspiring individuals through biographies, autobiographies, and memoirs. These stories can offer deep insights into how others have overcome obstacles and achieved their goals.

2. **Podcasts and Interviews:**

   - Listen to podcasts or watch interviews in which successful people share their journeys. Hearing their stories in their own words can provide relatable and actionable inspiration.

3. **Social Media:**

   - Follow people on platforms like Instagram, Twitter, or LinkedIn who share their experiences and advice. Social media allows you to connect with role models from various fields and industries.

4. **Local Community Groups:**

   - Engage with local community organizations, clubs, or volunteer groups where you can meet people who share your interests and values. Local leaders can serve as accessible and relatable role models.

5. **Mentorship Programs:**

   - Seek out formal mentorship programs in your industry or area of interest. Mentors can provide guidance and serve as role models based on their experience and success.

6. **Networking Events and Conferences**:

   - Attend industry conferences, workshops, or networking events where you can meet successful individuals who share your professional interests. These settings provide opportunities to connect with potential role models.

7. **Online Communities and Forums:**

   - Join online forums or communities related to your field or interests. These spaces can connect you with people who are further along in their journey and can serve as virtual role models.

8. **Friends and Family:**

   - Sometimes, the best role models are those closest to you. Friends, family members, or close acquaintances who have achieved something you admire can offer guidance and serve as relatable examples.

9. **Support Groups:**

   - Join a support group related to a challenge you're facing, whether it's related to health, addiction, or personal development. Role models in these groups can offer hope and strategies based on their experiences.

10. **Personal Development Workshops:**

- Participate in workshops or seminars focused on personal growth. The facilitators or fellow attendees can often become role models in your journey of self-improvement.

Finding your role model isn't about copying their path step for step. It's about seeing the possibilities they've created and realizing that you can create your own. It's about understanding that the only thing standing between you and your dreams is the belief that you can achieve them.

Now, go out and find your person. They're out there, living proof that your dreams aren't just fantasies—they're possibilities.

And if it's possible for them, it's possible for you too!

---

**Key Takeaways:**

- Role models are powerful because they show us what's possible. They inspire us to push through our fears and limitations.

- Finding and learning from role models can be a game changer in your journey toward achieving your goals.

## Questions:

1. How have role models impacted your belief in what's possible for you?

2. What steps will you take to seek out new role models who inspire you?

3. How can you become a role model for others who are facing similar challenges?

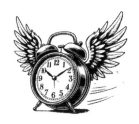

# CHAPTER 5: ESCALATE

## Small Actions, Big Impact

How do you win the Super Bowl?

Is it by beating the other team in the final game?

Well, yes. But not really. It's about much more than just that one big game. It's about every game that came before. Every practice session over the year. And every year before that. Each practice, each game, each pass caught or missed contributes to the final victory. Every single moment since you first played as a child.

Chances are you aren't dreaming of winning the Super Bowl. But the same idea applies to your dreams. All Dreams are a journey of immeasurable steps and efforts. It's not about one grand leap; it's about the accumulation of small victories and persistent efforts.

**Escalate** is that process of building over time. It

includes two main things:

1. **Building Bravery:** You want to know without question that you are someone who does hard things.
2. **Enhancing Expertise:** Having the skills to make your dream happen.

This combination is what allows you to truly know you are capable of doing the things needed to achieve your dreams.

Every time you do something hard, it gets easier the next time. But every time you give in to fear, the fear gets stronger.

You need to build your bravery to prove to yourself that you're someone who does hard things. You build bravery and expertise by doing hard things one step at a time, again and again. At each stage you will do a slightly bigger step into the scary to build your bravery and expertise.

Think of it like a staircase. You don't jump from the bottom to the top. You go step by step.

In this section, we will explore how to take those incremental steps to build your courage and resilience. By steadily escalating your efforts and confronting your fears, you will strengthen your ability to handle challenges and grow more confident in your capabilities. This process of escalation is crucial in proving to yourself that you can overcome obstacles and achieve your dreams, one step at a time.

---

**Key Takeaways:**

- Escalating your efforts gradually helps you build momentum without overwhelming yourself.

- Small, consistent actions lead to significant impacts over time, proving that you don't need to take massive leaps all at once to achieve big results.

**Questions:**

1. What small steps can you start taking today to escalate your efforts toward your goals?

2. What potential impact could these small, consistent actions have over time?

## A Story About Stabby Shells

One sunny afternoon in Ecuador, my parents, my husband Nabil, and I decided to take a long leisurely walk along the beach. We were in search of the most beautiful shells, and we had wandered to a spot where the shells were particularly sharp and spiky, yet undeniably stunning.

As we combed through the sand, I glanced at my watch. It showed that I had 40 minutes left before an important business call. I didn't think much of it until I realized that it had said 40 minutes the last time I checked as well. Panic set in as I realized my watch had stopped working. No one else had a phone or watch with them, so we had no idea what time it really was.

Panic set in. I had to get back. I started running, but the once-beautiful shells now felt like a bed of nails under my feet. Each step was agonizing, the sharp edges digging into my skin, but I couldn't stop. The physical pain was intense, but what was worse was the fear gnawing at me from the inside.

As I hopped and scrambled over the shells, it hit me that the pain wasn't just physical. Sure, my feet were hurting, but the deeper pain was the fear of what awaited me on that call. What if the client rejected me? What if I wasn't good enough? The easy way out would have been to stop, to use the shells as an excuse, to tell myself that there was no way I could make it back in time because of the "stabby" shells. It was a convenient out—a way to avoid facing the potential rejection that terrified me more than the physical pain.

But I knew that if I let the shells stop me, it wouldn't just be about missing the call. It would be about giving in to my fear, about letting that fear control my actions. So I kept going, pushing through the sharp stings beneath my feet and the even sharper doubts in my mind.

When I finally burst through the door of the house, I was a mess—disheveled, out of breath, and with only three minutes to spare. I jumped into the pool to cool off, trying to wash away the sweat and the fear. And then, with no time left to second-guess myself, I got on the call.

It wasn't just a call. It was a moment of reckoning when I had to decide whether I would let fear— physical or emotional—hold me back. And in that moment, I chose not to let it. I pushed through the pain, the fear, and the doubt, and I made that call.

And guess what?

I landed the client. The victory wasn't just in the

success of the call; it was in the decision to show up, despite the fear, despite the pain. The shells on the beach were just a distraction, a convenient excuse to give in to something deeper that was trying to stop me. But I didn't let it win. I chose to keep moving forward, no matter how hard or painful it felt at the time.

Because sometimes, the biggest obstacles aren't the ones under your feet—they're the ones in your mind. The only way to overcome them is to keep moving, one painful step at a time, until you get where you need to be.

---

**Key Takeaways:**

- The story of the stabby shells illustrates how fear and discomfort can tempt you to avoid challenging situations, but pushing through can lead to important achievements.

- It's essential to recognize when your fears are disguising themselves as physical discomfort to prevent you from reaching your goals.

**Questions:**

1. What situations have you faced in which pushing through the discomfort led to a significant achievement?

2. How can you better recognize when fear is disguised as something else and take action anyway?

# A Story About the Rule of 15

I used to underprice so badly that my first websites were priced for less than I now charge for one hour of time. Even as my skills and reputation grew, I continued to charge too little.

When it comes to achieving your goals—in both a personal and business context—practicality is key. I've promised you actionable, straightforward strategies that actually move the needle towards your dreams. The Rule of 15 is part of that.

While you may not be a business owner, you may have a side hustle or will consider one in the future. If not, I still recommend reading this short story, as there will be several non-business examples of how to use the Rule of 15 at the end of this section.

The tactic I am about to share is going to be game changing for you if you follow it.

Ready?

To make more money, you need to increase your prices.

It sounds simple, right? But if you've ever tried it, you know that the fear and hesitation that come with increasing prices can be paralyzing.

That's why I suggest a specific, systematic approach that I call Rule of 15 to make it less scary: you are going to incrementally increase your prices by 15% after selling something three times at your starting price.

- Then, you will sell it three times at the new price.
- Then, you increase the price by 15%.
- Sell it three more times.
- Increase by 15%
- Again and again and again; 15% every three sales.

And here's the crucial part—this isn't a suggestion you can flake on; it's a commitment you make to yourself. It's non-optional. By turning it into a rule, you take away the fear of making a decision each time. You've already decided that after three sales, the price goes up by 15%.

No debate, no second-guessing, just action.

This strategy is powerful because it minimizes the fear-induced paralysis associated with raising prices by providing a clear, manageable plan. You're not jumping into a huge price hike all at once;

you're taking calculated, incremental steps. Each increase is small enough that it feels achievable, yet significant enough that over time, it makes a real difference to your bottom line.

But let's be real—what if you raise your prices, and suddenly, you're truly finding it difficult to make sales? That's where the safety net comes in. If you truly hit a roadblock at the new price point, you have the option to step back to the previous price. But only do this once you have really tried to sell at the new price point. In my experience, most people will do many 15% increases before they hit major friction to sell at the newest price.

This method doesn't just help you overcome the fear of raising prices—it also establishes discipline. It helps you avoid the trap of self-sabotage, which I define as knowingly acting against your own best interests. The Terrorist in Your Head loves to provoke you into self-sabotage.

Implementing necessary steps towards your dream, like raising prices, takes courage. But courage doesn't mean you have to leap without a net. It means you have a plan—a practical, actionable plan that you follow through on, even when fear tries to get in the way. By systematically increasing your prices, you not only grow your business but also build your confidence in making tough decisions.

By deciding to commit to a *rule,* <u>you can mitigate your self-sabotage. The Rule gives you something to lean on.</u>

The Rule of 15 isn't just a business strategy; it's a life strategy. It's about making small, manageable changes or improvements that add up over time. These aren't just for your work life—they can be for anything that's important to you.

Imagine you've always wanted to learn a new language, but the idea of becoming fluent seems overwhelming. Instead of trying to master it all at once, apply the Rule of 15. Commit to learning just 15 new words or phrases each week. That's not a huge number—just a couple every day—but over the course of a year, you'll have learned over 750 words. That's enough to start having basic conversations and build your confidence.

Or consider your health. Maybe you want to start exercising, but you've never been able to stick with a routine. Start small—commit to just 15 minutes of movement each day. It doesn't have to be intense; it could be a walk, some stretching, or a short yoga session. By the end of the week, you'll have done nearly two hours of exercise. Over time, this small commitment builds into a habit that feels natural, not forced.

And what about your relationships? We often let small gestures of appreciation or love slip through the cracks of our busy lives. But what if you made it a rule to show your appreciation in 15 small ways each month? That could be as simple as leaving a note, sending a text, or doing something thoughtful for your loved ones. It doesn't take much time, but those small acts add up to a stronger, more connected relationship.

The Rule of 15 is powerful because it turns the overwhelming into the achievable. Whether it's in your career, your personal life, or your health, those incremental steps move you closer to your goals. And before you know it, those small efforts add up to big changes.

So, the next time you feel the hesitation creep in when it's time to take steps towards your dream, remember the Rule of 15. Commit to the rule, take the incremental steps, and trust the process.

---

**Key Takeaways:**

- Incremental changes will help you overcome the fear of fear of failing.
- Setting rules and sticking to them can alleviate the anxiety of decision-making and ensure

consistent progress.

**Questions:**

1. How can setting rules help you overcome fear and make better decisions?

2. What's one rule you can set for yourself today to help you move closer to your goals?

# A Story About Running in Circles

Every few years, when I would hit a plateau in my fitness training, I would get the idea that I wanted to run a marathon. I had never been a runner, but I had decent cardio from a childhood of being a gymnast. I hoped that working towards something big and impressive would re-motivate me to get more fit and stay fit long term.

...right?

Naturally, the first thing I did was download a bunch of training plans from the internet. You know, the ones with perfectly laid-out schedules that tell you exactly what to do every day for 12 weeks until you're crossing that finish line, victorious and glowing. I carefully amalgamated them, figuring out the one that seemed most reasonable. I was pumped. "Alright, 12 weeks to a marathon. I got this!" I thought.

I stuck to the plan perfectly on day one. Same for day two.

And then, on the third day, my knees hurt. Not a little bit of discomfort, but a real, nagging pain. So, I didn't run that day. And then the next day, I was stuck in this mental loop: "Do I skip today? Do I try to catch up? What do I do?" The indecision led to inaction, and of course, that spiraled into doing nothing at all.

Because that's what happens with those perfectly crafted, step-by-step plans—as soon as you miss a step or don't do it as well as you want, the fear of failure sneaks in. And suddenly, that fear becomes part of the process, and it's all downhill from there.

At this point, I was frustrated.

Here I was, knowing I was physically capable of running a marathon, but somehow I was letting the fear of messing up the plan derail everything. I realized that the plan itself, with all its meticulous details and timelines, was actually making it harder for me to just go out and do the thing.

So, I threw out all of the plans. I decided to just do it—no more overthinking, no more "what ifs."

All painful things are better with a friend, so I asked my most fit friend to do it with me. Always happy to have the opportunity to show off his physique, my friend agreed to join me that same day for a marathon.

So off we went to the track to run in circles for hours. I don't know how many laps we did, but it was a lot. A ridiculous amount of times. Around and around until we had done the distance as a marathon.

It was not fun. We only finished because we were

stubborn. And because we had told enough people that we were going to do this big thing that there had been people popping in to check on us all day. Quitting would be embarrassing. Social fears are powerful like that (and harnessing them is even more powerful!).

The next day, I felt like I was going to die. I tried to stand up, and my legs were screaming at me. I had never felt that kind of pain before—at least not at that age. But you know what? I did it. I didn't follow a perfect plan, I didn't train for 12 weeks straight, I didn't obsess over every little detail. I just decided to run, and I did it.

Sure, the time wasn't anything to write home about. In fact, we walked at least half of the time. Also, we ran indoors because I didn't want to deal with the weather—that was another potential excuse I knew would trip me up. But I finished. From finishing I realized two important things: first, I really was already physically capable of doing it. And second, I didn't actually want to do a marathon again. It was awful.

Also, to be clear, I do NOT recommend that particular approach to marathon running. I was already in great physical shape, and my body was used to taking a beating from years of cheerleading. For me, the block was entirely mental—that's where step one (DIAGNOSE) comes into play! I diagnosed my fear as mental, so I knew this approach would work.

The whole experience taught me that, sometimes, we get so caught up in making perfect plans that we paralyze ourselves with the fear of failing at them. But life isn't about sticking to some rigid plan. It's about knowing when to toss the plan out the window and just go for it. Sometimes, you have to ditch the meticulous preparation and simply see what happens. It might not be perfect, but at least it's done.

**Done is always better than perfect!**

Don't let the weight of creating a "perfect" plan hold you back. Sometimes, the best thing you can do is just start running—figuratively or literally—and trust that you'll figure it out as you go.

You might surprise yourself with what you're capable of, even if you never want to do it again.

---

**Key Takeaways:**

- Sometimes, elaborate plans can become overwhelming, leading to inaction. Simplifying your approach and just starting can be more effective.

- Achieving a goal doesn't always require perfect

execution; sometimes, just getting it done is what matters most.

## Questions:

1. What goals have you overcomplicated to the point of inaction?

2. How can you simplify your approach to these goals to make them more achievable?

# Conclusion on Escalate

When it comes to facing our fears, sometimes the best approach is to break them down into manageable pieces and tackle them with small, deliberate steps that get bigger as you go.

Here's a list of common fears and two small steps you can take to start overcoming them, all while staying aligned with the idea of diagnosing what's really holding you back.

---

## Fear of Public Speaking

- **Step 1:** Start by speaking up in small, informal settings, like team meetings or casual group discussions. Practice sharing your thoughts in a low-pressure environment to build confidence.

- **Step 2:** Record yourself speaking on a topic you're comfortable with. Play it back to get used to hearing your voice and refine your delivery without the immediate pressure of an audience.

---

## Fear of Networking or Meeting New People

- **Step 1:** Begin by attending small, local events where the stakes feel lower. Focus on having one meaningful conversation rather than trying to meet everyone.

- **Step 2:** Prepare a few simple conversation starters or questions in advance. Having these in your back pocket can ease the anxiety of breaking the ice with someone new.

---

## Fear of Failure

- **Step 1:** Reframe failure as feedback. Start with small tasks or projects in which the outcome isn't critical and use any mistakes as learning opportunities.

- **Step 2:** Set achievable, incremental goals that allow you to experience success more frequently. Celebrate these small wins to build momentum and confidence.

---

## Fear of Rejection

- **Step 1:** Practice asking for small things when a "no" won't have significant consequences—like asking for a favor from a colleague or a discount at a store. This helps desensitize you to rejection in low-stakes situations.

- **Step 2:** Keep a journal of positive interactions and outcomes to remind yourself that rejection isn't personal and that it doesn't define your worth.

## Fear of Sharing Your Work or Ideas

- **Step 1:** Start by sharing your work with a trusted friend or family member who will give you constructive feedback in a safe environment.

- **Step 2:** Post your work anonymously in an online forum or community that aligns with your interests. This allows you to receive feedback without the pressure of being personally identified.

## Fear of Change

- **Step 1:** Begin by making small, controlled changes in your daily routine, like taking a new route to work or trying a different type of food. This helps build your adaptability in a low-risk way.

- **Step 2:** Set short-term goals that require you to step slightly outside your comfort zone. Gradually increase the scale of these changes as you grow more comfortable with uncertainty.

## Fear of Making Decisions

- **Step 1:** Start with low-stakes decisions, like what to wear or what to eat for dinner, and make those choices quickly without second-guessing yourself.

- **Step 2:** Use a pros and cons list for more significant decisions. Limit yourself to a short amount of time to make a choice based on the information you have, rather than overanalyzing.

---

## Key Takeaways:

- Escalating your actions gradually allows you to build confidence and make meaningful progress without overwhelming yourself.

- Consistency and persistence are key to achieving long-term success, even if the steps seem small at the moment.

## Questions:

1. How can you apply the concept of escalation to your current goals?

2. How can you ensure that you keep escalating your efforts without giving up when it gets hard or scary?

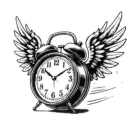

# CHAPTER 6: ALLY

## You Don't Need to Do This Alone

We all have moments when our confidence wavers, when that pesky Terrorist in Your Head creeps in, whispering doubts and feeding our insecurities. In those moments, it's easy to start questioning ourselves, our abilities, and our worth. That's where allies come in—those incredible people who believe in you and your potential even more than you do.

While you may be lucky enough to find a role model who is also your ally, that is most often not the case. You may never get to talk directly with your role models. Your allies however, are people who you will get close contact with and support from.

An ally is someone who sees the greatness in you, especially when you can't see it yourself. They're the ones who help you crumple up those paper dinosaurs and toss them aside. They remind you that you are smart, you are talented, you are confident, and you matter. Allies are the ones who stand by you, not just in the easy times, but especially when things get tough. They're the ones who tell you that you've got this, even when you're not so sure.

None of us can believe in ourselves a hundred percent of the time. It's just not possible. But with an ally by your side, those moments of doubt become smaller, more manageable. They help you remember who you are, what you're capable of, and why you're on this journey in the first place.

Let's explore the power of allies—the people who believe in us, fight for us, and stand with us as we face our fears and chase after our dreams. Because with the right allies, there's no limit to what we can achieve.

---

**Key Takeaways:**

- Allies are the people who believe in you even when you don't believe in yourself. They play a crucial role in helping you overcome challenges and achieve your goals.

- Surrounding yourself with the right allies can make all the difference in your journey toward success.

## Questions:

1. Who are your current allies, and how have they helped you in your journey?

2. How can you identify and cultivate new allies who believe in your potential?

3. What steps can you take to be a better ally to others in your life?

# A Story About See-Through Heels

There have been many times over the years that Lisa Larter has told me that I should do something far before I was ready. Writing this very book is an example of that. Lisa first told me I could and should do this six years before I said "yes" to my book publisher.

Speaking was another example of that. I had never considered speaking on stage before Lisa told me I should. At first, she casually mentioned that she was considering inviting a handful of regular business owners to share their stories at her next big event. It was January 2018, and the conference was 10 months away. Lisa had been my business strategist for just two months at this time. My business, Venture Creative Collective, was growing rapidly, and I had already completed four out of five of my ambitious goals for the year.

Because Lisa believed so much in me, it made me willing to try to earn a spot, but... who was I to think that Lisa would choose me? Lots of people would surely apply for this opportunity. Besides, I'd never spoken on a stage before! Heck, I didn't even want to be a speaker! Yet, the draw to be on that stage remained, persistent and compelling.

I was thinking about this while surfing the internet,

window shopping on a fancy shoe website.

Then, I saw them. The coolest shoes ever.

The moment I saw them, I knew the unique transparent heels were meant for the stage. Wearing them on a stage would make me look like I was floating! The illusion of floating captivated me, and yet, I almost passed them over. *"I have no reason to buy those shoes,"* I told myself. *"I can't buy them with the assumption that I will get chosen. It will be so embarrassing if I don't."*

In our first call, Lisa told me that success comes to those who are willing to be uncomfortable. *"Success lives on the other side of fear,"* she said. *"What would you do if you weren't afraid?"*

Lisa's words echoed in my mind as I stared at those transparent heels. She wanted me to speak. She told me about the opportunity. She encouraged me to apply. She believed in me.

*"Add to cart."*

I told no one, not even Lisa, when I bought them. I said nothing when the box arrived in the mail. And certainly not over the coming months when the "stage heels" sat untouched on the shelf, challenging me to prove I had a story worth sharing with 400 people. Every time I glanced at them, they whispered to me, reminding me of my unspoken desire to conquer the stage.

Ten months later, my audacious goal became reality. I was standing in front of that audience, wearing those transparent heels, and I felt a mix of nerves and exhilaration. As I shared my story, I realized that this moment was not just about me; it was about everyone who has ever doubted their potential. It was about stepping out of my comfort zone and embracing the fear of the unknown.

That question has guided me through many decisions, but never as profoundly as it did with those transparent heels. They were more than just shoes; they were a symbol of my willingness to take risks, to dream big, and to push through my fears. My advisor, Lisa Larter, provided the stage and the encouragement, but I had to do the work to earn a spot on it.

Now, I ask you the same question:

*"What would you do if you weren't afraid?"*

Decide what that is. Then find an ally to support your dreams, take the risk, and buy those metaphorical heels. Success truly does live on the other side of fear.

**Key Takeaways:**

- Having someone in your corner who believes in you can push you to take risks and achieve things you never thought possible.

- Allies can help you see past your fears and encourage you to step into opportunities with confidence.

**Questions:**

1. Do you have an ally in your life who will push you to take risks and seize opportunities, even before you see them as possible for yourself?

2. What item could you pre-purchase as a symbol of the dream you are trying to reach? Who could you tell about that item so they can support your dream?

# A Story About A Platform

In Chapter 4, I told you about how I started speaking regularly on stages.

The potential to be a role model was a powerful motivator, but it wasn't the most significant one. The real driving force behind my journey into public speaking was the desire to be an ally for those, like me, who live with narcolepsy.

Narcolepsy is a condition that often takes 10 to 15 years to diagnose from the time symptoms first appear. Imagine that—over a decade of suffering, confusion, and misdiagnosis before finally getting the answers you need. I was fortunate enough to have a friend, Becky, who saw the signs in me and pushed me toward getting the help I needed. Her insistence saved me years of frustration and hardship.

But not everyone with narcolepsy is so lucky.

That's where I saw the opportunity to make a difference. I realized that if I could share my story on the biggest stages, if I could become a speaker recognized for her impact and reach, I might be able to shorten that diagnostic journey for even one person. If just one person in those audiences saw answers for themselves or someone they know from hearing my story and sought help sooner because of it, it could change their life entirely.

Narcolepsy is rare, and the people who need to hear my story are scattered across the globe. That's why I set an ambitious goal: to speak on 100 stages in two years. I knew that to reach the level of influence I aspired to, I needed to put in the reps. I needed to escalate my efforts, build my skills, and get in front of as many people as possible as quickly as possible.

These reps weren't just about telling my story the same way again and again—it was about refining it, amplifying it, and making it resonate on a level that could truly make a difference. I was driven by the knowledge that my words could save someone years of unnecessary suffering. That's why I committed to this goal with everything I had. Because if I could help even one person get diagnosed sooner, if I could save them five years of their life, it would all be worth it.

And that's why I speak. That's why I push myself to reach higher, to be better, and to stand on those stages—100 of them in two years. It's about more than just sharing; it's about creating real, meaningful change.

Within the first 10 stages, something profound happened.

A young woman came up to me at the end of the

event and said, *"Can I speak to you privately?"*

The emotion in her voice was causing every word to shake as it came out.

*"I have never seen someone with a service dog in a professional business setting before."*
*"I tried to come to your session today, but the room was already full. So I Googled you instead."*
*"Has having a service dog ruined your career? It doesn't look like it has from Google."*

With every sentence her emotion got stronger.

It turned out she had an invisible disability and had been training a service dog at home.

But no one knew outside of her doctor and family. Until that moment.

*How familiar is that story?!*

We spent the next 15 minutes talking about my story and how I had the same worries before being publicly *"out"* about having a disability.

By the end, there was no longer shaking in her voice, and instead she was smiling.

*"I am so glad I saw you today. This has changed everything for me. I am not afraid anymore."*

At that moment, it was no longer her who was overcome with emotion.

THIS is the reason I set a goal of speaking on 100 stages within two years.

Very, very few people who see me speak or meet me at big events will have narcolepsy like I do.

But many will have "something."

I thought I would have to speak on 100 stages to be "big enough" to be able to have moments like this.

I was wrong.

Every stage is an opportunity to make a difference. I have the potential to provide guidance, advice, and encouragement to people who come to listen to my story. I can be both a role model and an ally to them.

I bet there is someone in your life that you could do the same for.

I have no doubts that once I meet and exceed the 100 stages goal, even more incredible things will happen. But I am also appreciative of everything that is happening along the way.

---

## Key Takeaways:

- The next time you are at an event, take a deeper look at the people who are there to see if there is a potential ally for you.
- By being vulnerable and asking for help, you could get the answers you need to move forward towards your dream.

## Questions:

1. How can you use your own experiences to inspire and support others facing similar challenges?
2. Who in your life might benefit from hearing your story?

# A Story About a Not-So Blue Dress

One of the most wonderful things about having an ally is that they see your potential, even when you're trying to talk yourself out of it. They're there to push you forward, to remind you that you can do it, and to be the support you need when the pressure is on.

Let me tell you a story about my niece, Runa. Quinn, my current narcolepsy service dog, also happens to be a Canadian Grand Champion show dog, thanks to my husband Nabil, who is her handler. We've spent countless weekends at dog shows to earn that title, and along the way, our family often came to cheer us on. Runa, my brother's oldest child, was one of our most enthusiastic supporters.

Runa was captivated by the dog shows. One day, at the age of five, she came to me, eyes wide with determination, and said, *"Michelle, I wanna be like Nabil and run around in a circle with a dog for that man in a suit!"*

Word for word, that's what she said.

I couldn't help but smile and say, *"Okay, let's figure out how to make this happen."*

We discovered that kids could indeed participate in dog shows, and we found a more size-appropriate dog than our towering Great Dane. When the day of her first show arrived, Runa was excited, but she was also incredibly nervous. As much as she wanted to be like her Uncle Nabil, that first step into the ring was a big one.

Despite having been very excited for weeks leading up to the big show day, nervous doesn't even begin to describe how she felt as the moment to enter the ring got closed. Five minutes before showtime, she looked up at the nice lady whose small dog she was borrowing and said with big, anxious eyes, *"I can't do the dog show today..."*

*"Why not, sweetie?"*

*"Well... my dress is not blue enough."*

There it was—a classic excuse—the fear dressed up as something entirely unrelated to the task at hand. And as I looked into her face, I realized how universal that feeling is. We've all been there, trying to pull that kind of excuse on ourselves when we're scared to take the leap.

But that's where an ally steps in.

Her ally bent down to Runa's level, took her hands, and talked her through it. They didn't dismiss her fear; instead, they acknowledged it and worked with it. They offered to get her a balloon on a leash for Runa to practice with, helping her get comfortable with the motions before stepping into the ring with a dog.

And you know what happened next?

Runa walked into that ring, held onto that leash, and did exactly what she set out to do. She even won first place! Although, as she will proudly tell you, *"All the other kids won first place too!"*

But the real victory was Runa overcoming her nerves and doing the thing she was so scared to do but had been dreaming of. That wouldn't have happened without an ally who believed in her, who knew what she was capable of, even when she wasn't so sure herself.

That's the power of having someone in your corner— someone who will help you practice with balloons when your dress isn't blue enough and who will talk you through the moments when you want to turn and run.

Allies aren't just there to cheer you on; they're there to stand beside you, to guide you, and to help you realize that you can do the very thing you're afraid of. They don't let you quit on your dreams.

**Key Takeaways:**

- Allies can provide the support and encouragement needed to push through moments of self-doubt.

- Having someone to lean on in difficult moments can be the difference between giving up and moving forward.

**Questions:**

1. When was the last time an ally helped you overcome a moment of self-doubt?

2. What challenges are you facing that could be easier to overcome with the help of an ally?

# Conclusion on Ally

Having an ally isn't just a nice thing—it's crucial.

I have had the extreme privilege of having two parents, David and Evelyn Weger, who have both been great allies throughout my life.

My dad, the military man, often took longer to warm up to my more unconventional ideas, but is always there when I call him to ask for a helping hand. From helping me to move many times to rush-building a closet with me when I wanted to surprise Nabil but got in over my head, if he can physically come help then he will.

My mom, the social worker, never hesitated to support any of my ideas. My dad was away for months each year on military work. Despite how hard that must have been for her, my mom always gave enough support and love for two parents.

We moved every two years, as military families often do. There were many years when I did not have friends, but I never felt deeply alone, thanks in large part to my parents.

They have both shown up for me through my whole life. I know that is not the case for many, if not most, people.

I have several friends who do not have a positive

relationship with one or both of their own parents. My mom, Evelyn, is there for those friends, who call her when they need a mom to talk to. She is always chiming in on social media to congratulate the people who matter to me on their accomplishments. Talk about the ultimate ally!

I truly hope that each of you has at least one person like this in your life.

You deserve it. You deserve someone who lifts you up, who believes in your potential, and who helps you navigate through the doubts and fears that inevitably arise. And if you don't have that person right now, know that you're not alone, and there are people out there who will believe in you.

Please, reach out—to me, to others—and let's find someone who will be that unwavering support for you.

Join my DREAM community to find and be a role model or ally: https://michelleweger.com/dream-community/

## Key Takeaways:

- Allies are essential to overcoming the challenges and fears that hold you back. They provide the support, encouragement, and belief in your potential that you might not always have yourself.

- Building strong relationships with allies can help you achieve your goals more effectively and with greater confidence.

## Questions:

1. How can you strengthen your relationships with your current allies?

2. Who in your life could benefit from your support as an ally?

3. What steps will you take to ensure you have a strong network of allies to help you on your journey?

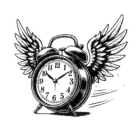

# CHAPTER 7: MEMORIALIZE

## Building Confidence for When the Bad Things Actually Happen

We all have fears. Those nagging, persistent worries that sit in the back of our minds. But what do you do when the bad things you are afraid will happen actually do happen? How do you cope when your fears materialize right before your eyes?

I've always been a big believer in facing fears head-on. But let's be real—sometimes it's not that simple. Our brains are wired to focus on negative outcomes as a protective measure. This tendency can make it challenging to move forward when things go wrong.

*How many times has one negative comment drowned out 10 positive ones?*

However, there are strategies to counteract this natural inclination.

One approach I find incredibly effective is

acknowledging and celebrating successes. It's easy to get caught up in the negative, but keeping a record of positive outcomes or "wins" can provide a much-needed perspective shift. For instance, if someone criticizes your pricing—something many of us fear—you can look at a folder filled with accepted estimates. This concrete evidence shows that the criticism is an outlier, not the norm. It's a powerful way to remind your brain that success is far more common than failure.

Think about it: you receive a stinging piece of feedback about your prices being too high. That fear of not being good enough, or of not offering value, suddenly feels very real. But then you open your folder of accepted estimates and see proof of your worth. It's a visual and emotional reminder that the negative feedback is just one piece of the puzzle. It doesn't define your entire business or your worth.

This method isn't just about countering negativity; it's about building a mental toolkit that helps you stay focused on your goals. When things go wrong, and they inevitably will, you need strategies in place to help you push through. Documenting your successes is one such strategy. It's not about denying the bad but about giving yourself a balanced view when The Terrorist in Your Head tries to gaslight you.

Even if you're tackling something new and don't have direct proof of success in that area, you can draw confidence from your other achievements. Your past successes in different areas can provide the boost you need to tackle new challenges with confidence. This approach helps keep your brain from reverting to a fearful state, showing it that you are capable of overcoming obstacles.

It's also important to recognize that our brains lean towards the negative as a means of protection. Understanding this can help us rationalize our fears. When something bad happens, it's natural to focus on it. But by acknowledging this tendency, we can consciously shift our focus to the positive evidence we've accumulated.

Let's face it: life is full of stabby shells. There will be moments when you feel like you're running over sharp obstacles, trying to reach your goals. But just like my experience running across the beach in Ecuador, sometimes you have to endure immediate discomfort to achieve long-term success. The pain is temporary, but the success that comes from pushing through it is lasting.

So, what do you do when bad things actually happen? You keep going. You pull out your folder of wins and remind yourself of all the times you succeeded. You let those successes drown out the negative voices.

And you push through the pain, knowing that on the other side lies the success you're working so hard to achieve.

In life and business, setbacks are inevitable. But with the right strategies, you can overcome them. Celebrate your wins, document your successes, and use them as a buffer against the bad. Lean on proof of your abilities and tenacity to keep running, even when it hurts, because the rewards on the other side are always well worth the effort.

---

## Key Takeaways:

- Memorializing your successes helps build confidence and serves as a reminder of your progress, especially when facing new challenges.
- Creating tangible reminders of your achievements can motivate you to keep pushing forward and set new goals.

## Questions:

1. What successes have you achieved that you can memorialize to build confidence?
2. How can you create tangible reminders of your progress to keep yourself motivated?

# A (Different) Story About Dog Shows

As adults, we don't often get physical tokens of our achievements. The little things that say, *"Hey, you did great today!"* seem to fade away after we leave childhood behind. We don't get gold stars for a job well done at work, and no one hands out medals for making it through a tough week. But I've found something that brings back that feeling of being rewarded for hard work: dog show ribbons.

If you've ever been to a dog show, you know that ribbons are a big deal. They're not just for the dogs—they're for the handlers and owners too. They're a tangible, colorful reminder of the effort, the training, and the countless hours spent working toward a goal.

And they feel good to get. Really good. Because, let's face it, we all need those moments when someone—or something—says, *"You did it. You were the best today."*

One of my proudest moments came when Quinn won the ribbon for Best of Opposite (meaning Female Great Dane) in the entire speciality dog show. Now, if you've ever seen a Great Dane up close, you know they're not exactly small dogs. That should give you an idea of how huge that ribbon is; it is taller than a Great Dane!

There's something deeply satisfying about being handed a ribbon. It's more than just a strip of fabric. It's validation. It's recognition of all the hard work, the early mornings, the endless training sessions. And it's something I think we could all use a little more of in our lives.

Why don't we, as adults, get more of these kinds of affirmations?

Why don't we have more ways to celebrate our wins, big or small?

Maybe we should.

Maybe we should give ourselves ribbons, or the adult equivalent—whether it's treating ourselves to something special after a big achievement or simply taking a moment to acknowledge our progress. It's important to have those reminders, those little rewards that say, *"You're doing great. Keep going."*

Each of the ribbons I've collected over the years tells a story of a challenge faced, a goal met, a moment of triumph. And every time I look at them, I'm reminded of the journey I've taken with Quinn and Max before her. They are more than just decorations—they're milestones of our shared success, proof of our hard work, and they make me feel good every time I see them.

Whether it's a ribbon, a certificate, or just a mental

high-five, find a way to celebrate your wins. Because we all deserve a little something to remind us of how far we've come.

---

## Key Takeaways:

- Celebrating your achievements, no matter how big or small, is essential for building confidence and recognizing your progress.

- Tangible rewards, like ribbons from dog shows, serve as powerful reminders of what you've accomplished.

## Questions:

1. What smaller achievements in your life deserve to be celebrated and memorialized?

2. How can you create tangible reminders of these achievements to keep yourself motivated?

# A Story About Jimmy Choo Sneakers

*"What is celebrated is repeated."*

I am, admittedly, a competitive person. I'm always looking to "beat" myself month-over-month and year-over-year. This drive for constant improvement means I often focus too much energy on my shortcomings and mistakes. It comes naturally to me to overlook my accomplishments, even when things are going exceptionally well.

In an effort to combat this mentality, I decided to celebrate my big milestones in 2018 by treating myself to a pair of shoes every time I met my goals for any given month. This practice was a deliberate attempt to shift my focus from what went wrong to what went right. It forced me to acknowledge and celebrate the good things I wanted to see happen again and again.

At the beginning of the year, my shoe closet was relatively sparse, with a few trusty pairs that had seen better days. As the months went by and I started hitting my targets, the shelves began to fill up with increasingly unique and stylish heels. Each new pair was a tangible reminder of my hard work and success. It was more motivating than I had ever expected.

When I exceeded my income goal for 2018 a month

early, I knew I had to celebrate with a particularly special pair of shoes. I started browsing online, and that's when I stumbled upon the sparkly "Miami" Jimmy Choo sneakers. They were dazzling, a real statement piece.

But then the doubts crept in... Could I? ... Should I? ... Would I?

The idea of owning those shoes was thrilling, but I hesitated. Was it too extravagant? Was I being frivolous?

However, deep down, I knew that these shoes were more than just a purchase. They were a symbol of my hard-earned success and a testament to my dedication and perseverance.

In the end, the answer was undeniable. Of the 12+ varieties of Jimmy Choo sneakers online, the only style available in my size at the store in Florida were those Miami shoes! It felt like fate. I walked out of the store with a bounce in my step and a grin that wouldn't quit.

This journey taught me a valuable lesson. Too often, we focus on what needs to be fixed or improved, losing sight of our achievements along the way. By refocusing on the successes in your life, not only will you feel better about yourself, but you'll also find that you succeed more often and at a higher level.

So, I challenge you to celebrate your milestones, no matter how small. Whether it's a new pair of shoes or another treat that brings you joy, find a way to acknowledge your victories. Because what is celebrated is repeated. And trust me, it feels fantastic to watch your accomplishments pile up, one fabulous pair of shoes at a time.

---

**Key Takeaways:**

- Rewarding yourself for reaching milestones can be a powerful motivator and a way to recognize your hard work.

- Treating yourself to something special after achieving a goal reinforces the positive behavior and encourages you to keep going.

**Questions:**

1. What milestones have you reached recently that deserve a reward?

2. What reward can you plan for yourself once you reach your next big milestone?

# A Story About a Supercar

As you know, there was a time when I wasn't allowed to drive. A medical suspension from narcolepsy had taken away my right to get behind the wheel, and with it, a piece of my independence. But when I finally earned back that right, I made a promise to myself: if I was going to drive again, I was going to *drive*. When I was able to buy a second car, I wasn't just going to get any car—I was going to get a car that symbolizes overcoming not just the medical challenges, but the financial limits that so many people with narcolepsy face.

I started dreaming about it, browsing through cars online, imagining myself in something sporty, fun, and undeniably cool. I kept coming back to Lotus cars—the Elise and the Exige. They're just so sporty, so fast, so everything I wanted my driving experience to be. They are also similar to a go kart in the sense that they are built to be as light as possible so they can be extra fast. There is little seat padding, and the passenger window doesn't even open without a hand crank!

Between the dreaming and the day I made the first purchase, I met someone very special: Nabil Ould-Brahim. We met playing flag football and quickly realized we were both very goal-oriented people. We began meeting up for coworking sessions, where we openly shared our goals and what we had accomplished since our last meeting.

Nabil is the smartest man I have ever met. He encouraged me to go after all my dreams, no matter how difficult or distant they seemed. I did the same for him. We were open and honest with each other, sharing both the good and the bad on our paths to making our dreams come true. Nabil was the first man, outside of my father, with whom I could truly be myself. He accepted me as I was, narcolepsy included, and wanted to know all of me—not just the flashy, public-facing parts. I felt the same way about him.

We even shared a dream. We both wanted a supercar one day!

After being friends and allies to each other for nine months, we went on our first date. Our wedding was exactly one year from that first date. *When you know, you know!*

When the time came to make our shared car dream a reality, Nabil and I ended up choosing something a bit more understated, but infinitely more luxurious than my original idea: an Aston Martin V8 Vantage. It wasn't just a car—it was a statement.

That car was more than just a purchase. It was a symbol of everything we had achieved, both individually and together. It was about reclaiming something I had lost and proving that limits, whether medical or financial, are only temporary when you're determined enough to push past them.

Of course, living in Canada means the car spends half the year in storage, waiting out the long, cold winter. It's not the most practical car by any means, but that was never the point.

Every spring, when we finally take it out for the first drive of the year, I still get teary-eyed with gratitude and amazement the first time I hit the gas on a long stretch and feel all the power of that engine. The symbolism hits me deep. Every single time.

I think back to the days when driving wasn't even an option for me, and here I am, behind the wheel of a car that represents so much more than just transportation. It's a reminder that with hard work and perseverance, you can take back what was taken from you—and even more.

---

**Key Takeaways:**

- Earning a big, physical memorialization is as much about recognizing the journey and hard work that got you there as the material reward itself.

- Large, tangible symbols of success can serve

as reminders of what you've overcome and achieved over a long period of time.

## Questions:

1. What large, tangible symbols of success do you have in your life that remind you of your achievements?

2. What's the huge reward you're working toward, and how will it symbolize your hard work and success?

## Conclusion on Memorialize

It's easy to get caught up in the day-to-day grind and forget to celebrate the wins—both big and small—that got you where you are today. But these moments deserve to be remembered and cherished, not just for the joy they bring, but for the confidence they can instill when those paper dinosaurs come creeping back.

Here are some ideas to help you celebrate your successes and keep them front and center in your life:

**1. Evidence Folder:**

- Create a folder where you save printed emails, thank you notes, or testimonials from clients, colleagues, or anyone who has recognized your good work. When you're feeling unsure or doubting yourself, open it up and remind yourself of all the positive impact you've made.

**2. Drawer of Appreciation:**

- Dedicate a drawer or a box to store cards, letters, or little tokens of appreciation from people who value you. These physical reminders can be incredibly uplifting, especially on tough days.

## 3. Ribbon Wall:

- If you've won awards, completed significant milestones, or even participated in events that matter to you, display those ribbons, medals, or certificates on a wall. Seeing them every day is a powerful reminder of what you're capable of.

## 4. Photo Folder on Your Phone:

- Create a special album on your phone for photos that make you proud—whether it's of work you've done, events you've participated in, or moments when you felt truly accomplished. It's a portable reminder of your journey and growth.

## 5. Share Your Wins with Allies:

- Don't keep your successes to yourself—share them with your allies. Whether it's over coffee, in a group chat, or during a casual catch-up, let the people who support you know about your achievements. Remember, telling the truth about your success isn't bragging; it's owning your journey and recognizing your worth.

## 6. Success Journal:

- Keep a dedicated journal where you write down your accomplishments, no matter how small. Reflect on what you did, how you felt, and why it mattered. Over time, this journal becomes a personal record of your growth and achievements.

## 7. Achievement Tokens:

- Collect small tokens or mementos that represent your successes—like a special pen, a piece of jewelry, or a figurine. Display them in a spot where you can see them regularly as a physical reminder of what you've accomplished.

## 8. Social Media Highlights:

- Use your social media profiles to create highlight reels or albums that showcase your achievements. It's a way to share your successes with others while also creating a digital archive of your milestones.

## 9. Success Jar:

- Keep a jar on your desk or in your home, and every time you achieve something, write it on a piece of paper and drop it in the jar. At the end of the year (or whenever you need a boost), read through the notes to see just how much you've accomplished.

## 10. Create a Personal Trophy:

- Design a custom trophy or plaque for yourself, and add to it each time you achieve something significant. It might seem a bit quirky, but it's a fun and tangible way to celebrate your wins.

Success isn't just about reaching the finish line; it's about acknowledging and celebrating each step along the way.

By memorializing these moments, you create a reservoir of confidence and positivity that you can draw from whenever you need a boost. It's a way to honor your hard work and remind yourself that you're capable of greatness, even when those pesky doubts try to tell you otherwise.

---

## Key Takeaways:

- Memorializing your successes helps solidify your achievements and provides motivation for future challenges.
- Tangible reminders of your progress, whether they're physical objects or mental milestones, can keep you focused and driven.

## Questions:

1. Have you memorialized your successes in the past? How can you do it more intentionally moving forward?

2. What achievements are you most proud of, and how can you keep them top of mind?

3. How can you use your past successes as fuel for achieving even greater things in the future?

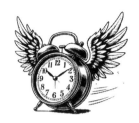

# CONCLUSION: A STORY ABOUT OWNING YOUR JOURNEY

As we reach the end of this book, I want to take a moment to remind you of something important: this is your journey. Every fear you face, every step you take, every win you celebrate—it's all uniquely yours. We've talked about overcoming fears, about finding your allies and role models, and about the importance of memorializing your successes. But at the heart of all of this is the simple truth that your path is yours to create, navigate, and own.

When I started this journey, I had no idea where it would take me. I didn't plan to become a speaker, or a business owner, or a champion of anything, really. I was just trying to figure out how to live my life with narcolepsy, to find a way to be successful on my own terms. But along the way, I discovered that the challenges I faced, the fears I had to confront, and the victories I celebrated weren't just about me—they were about all of us who are trying to do something big with our lives.

This book isn't about telling you that you have to conquer every fear or be the best at everything you do. It's about recognizing that you have the power to choose what matters to you. It's about understanding that you don't have to face every fear—just the ones that are holding you back from what you truly want. It's about knowing that sometimes, it's okay to walk away from something that doesn't serve you, and it's more than okay to celebrate the things that do.

Throughout these chapters, I've shared stories of how I've faced my own fears, found my own role models, and built my own tribe of allies. I've talked about the power of small steps and the importance of taking action, even when it's scary. But most of all, I've tried to show you that your life—your journey—is something worth investing in, worth fighting for, and worth celebrating.

As you close this book, I want you to remember that you are capable of more than you know. Whatever your DREAM is, I know that you have what it takes to make it happen.

And when you do, don't forget to take a moment to acknowledge how far you've come. Celebrate your wins, no matter how small they might seem.

Memorialize them, because they are proof that you are moving forward, that you are growing, and that you are living a life that is truly yours.

Thank you for sharing this journey with me.

I hope that as you move forward, you continue to face your fears, find your allies, and create a life that makes you proud. Because at the end of the day, that's what it's all about—living a life that's true to who you are and knowing that you have the power to make it as amazing as you want it to be.

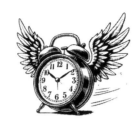

# APPENDICES

## A Poem About Narcolepsy

**By Rebecca Bodnar**

I have this inner demon, and she
is living right inside of me.
She steals my waking moments, then
she spits them back at me again.
Twists them while I writhe in sleep,
When suddenly I slumber deep.
I take a pill, she quiets down,
Though she will forever be around.
My body like a prison cell
has almost certainly seen hell.
I owe it to myself to fight,
To turn the darkness into light.
She knows that I am easily mired,
Not much strength left in the tired.
But she's shown me where to find
A fighter of a different kind.
And though she's still the enemy

Somehow she's been a friend to me
Teaching me what can't be taught
Giving me what can't be bought
To lend an empathetic ear
To understand and conquer fear
To tell myself that I am strong
As she whispers "no, you're wrong"
To always take it day by day
And seldom let her have her way.

# Key Takeaways

In this section, I've distilled the essence of the book into key takeaways. These are the core lessons and strategies that I hope you will carry with you:

- **Embrace Your Unique Story:** Your challenges and experiences are a source of strength and authenticity.

- **Recognize and Name Your Fears:** Understanding your fears is the first step to overcoming them.

- **Small Acts of Bravery Lead to Greatness:** Courage is built through consistent, small steps outside your comfort zone.

- **Celebrate Every Success:** Acknowledging and celebrating your achievements fosters a positive mindset and motivation.

- **Physical Reminders of Success Are Powerful:** Tangible representations of your achievements can be a continual source of inspiration.

- **Seek and Be an Ally:** Building relationships with mentors and being a mentor to others is invaluable for growth.

- **Action Overcomes Fear:** Knowledge is powerful, but action is transformative.

- **Resilience Is Key:** The ability to bounce back and learn from challenges is essential for long-term success.

- **Your Potential Is Boundless:** Never underestimate your ability to grow, adapt, and achieve.

# DREAM Method by Michelle Weger

## 1. <u>Diagnose</u>: Recognize and Name Your Fears

- Key Insight: Identifying what you're afraid of is the first step in overcoming fear.

- Action: Write down your fears to acknowledge them. This process demystifies fears and reduces their hold over you.

- Key Insight: Most fears are more psychological than physical, often rooted in judgment or failure.

- Action: Analyze each fear to understand its origin. Ask yourself: "Is this fear rational? Will it truly harm me?"

## 2. <u>Role Model</u>: Seek Inspiration From People "Like You" Who Have Achieved Something Great

- Key Insight: Seeing others overcome similar fears and barriers can be incredibly motivating.

- Action: Research and read stories about people who have faced and conquered fears similar to yours and/or who have similar challenges, life experiences, or backgrounds to yours who have done great things.

## 3. <u>Escalate</u>: Start with Small Challenges, Build Up

- Key Insight: Action is the most effective counter to fear.

- Action: Implement the plans you have made, even if it's a small step. Remember, action builds momentum.

- Key Insight: Courage is built through consistent, small acts of bravery.

- Action: Set small, achievable challenges for yourself that push you slightly out of your comfort zone.

- Key Insight: Discipline and resilience are key in facing and overcoming challenges.

- Action: Engage in activities that require discipline, like the 75 Hard Challenge, to build resilience.

## 4. <u>Ally</u>: Find an Ally to Support Your Journey

- Key Insight: Allies, mentors, and supporters can provide guidance and encouragement.

- Action: Seek out allies (and become one for others).

- Key Insight: Your unique experiences, including challenges, are a source of strength and authenticity.

- Action: Share your story with others. This not only empowers you but can also inspire others.

## 5. <u>Memorialize</u>: Celebrate Your Successes

- Key Insight: Acknowledging and celebrating achievements bolsters confidence and reinforces a positive mindset.

- Action: Create physical reminders of your successes, such as mementos or a success journal.

# About The Author

Michelle Weger is a dynamic entrepreneur, speaker, and advocate who has built a successful career on the foundation of resilience, creativity, and determination. As the founder and CEO of Venture Creative Collective (VCC), Michelle has built a highly regarded website development and business automation business that has helped hundreds of countless businesses streamline their processes and achieve remarkable growth. Known for her innovative approach, Michelle has garnered praise for her company's unique "Website in a Day" service, which delivers fully customized websites in record time.

A trailblazer in her field, Michelle's expertise extends beyond just business. She has been featured on platforms like CBC Marketplace and "You Can't Ask That," sharing her insights and experiences with a broader audience. Her commitment to inclusivity and accessibility in business is deeply personal, as Michelle has lived with narcolepsy, a disabling lifelong sleep disorder, since her early twenties. This diagnosis has fueled her passion for advocacy, leading her to raise awareness about narcolepsy and accessibility for others living with disabilities.

Michelle's story is not just about overcoming

obstacles—it's about embracing them and turning them into opportunities. Whether she's mentoring other entrepreneurs, developing new tools for business automation, or speaking on stages across the globe, Michelle's message is clear: no matter the challenges you face, you can still achieve your dreams.

Michelle's journey wouldn't be complete without acknowledging the unwavering support of her husband, Nabil Ould-Brahim. Nabil is not only her business partner but also her rock and her biggest champion. His incredible intellect, constant encouragement, and steadfast love make him the best husband she could ever ask for. Together, they've built a life and a business that reflect their shared values of innovation, integrity, and relentless pursuit of excellence.

In addition to her business ventures, Michelle is an avid traveler, adventurer, and animal lover. She is one of the first people in the world with a Great Dane service dog for narcolepsy. Her current service dog, Quinn, is not only a Grand Champion show dog but also participates in dock diving and agility competitions. Michelle's life is a testament to the idea that you don't have to choose between passion and practicality—you can have both.

Michelle lives life on her own terms, always striving to push the boundaries of what's possible. Whether she's in the boardroom, on the stage, or training with Quinn, Michelle Weger is a force to be reckoned with—proof that with the right mindset and tools, anything is possible.

- Instagram: @daneonaplane
- TikTok: @adaneonaplane
- Website: www.michelleweger.com/
- Email: michelle@venturecreative.com
- More links: www.michelleweger.com/links/

*thank you*

# THANK YOU
# FOR READING MY BOOK!

Dear Reader,

Well, you made it to the end—congrats! I hope you found some insights, a few laughs, and maybe even a bit of inspiration along the way. Sharing these stories and lessons has been a real adventure, and I'm thrilled you chose to spend your time with me.

Now, I need your help!

If you found value in these pages (or if you just really like dogs and success stories), I'd love it if you could take a minute to leave a **5-star review on Amazon**. Not only will it make my day, but it'll also help this book reach more people who could benefit from it. Think of it as a little ripple effect—your review could be the nudge someone needs to pick up the book and start making changes in their own life.

Thanks so much!

Michelle

# Additional Resources

- Narcolepsy Network. (2016). Narcolepsy and Employment Survey. Retrieved from narcolepsynetwork.org

- Jennum, P., Ibsen, R., Knudsen, S., & Kjellberg, J. (2012). The economic consequences of narcolepsy: a controlled national study of patients and their spouses. *Sleep*, 35(6), 667-672.

- Pizza, F., Moghadam, K. K., Vandi, S., Detto, S., Poli, F., Franceschini, C., & Mignot, E. (2013). Narcolepsy with cataplexy: hypocretin receptor 2 gene mutation in a family with multiple cases. *Sleep*, 36(6), 833-838.

- Broughton, W. A., & Broughton, R. J. (1994). Psychosocial impact of narcolepsy. *Sleep*, 17(8), S45-S49.

- Thorpy, M., & Dauvilliers, Y. (2016). Diagnosis, evaluation, and management of narcolepsy: an update. *Sleep Medicine Reviews*, 29, 21-32.

- Startup Unicorns - Link

- https://onlinelibrary.wiley.com/doi/full/10.1111/jsr.14087

# MY GIFT TO YOU

As a special thank you for reading, I'm excited to offer you FREE access to my VIP email list, where I share exclusive surprise bonuses.

You'll receive free coloring sheets as an immediate gift. In Chapter 3, I discuss how taking small steps, like coloring without fear of judgment, can help build the confidence needed to tackle life's bigger challenges.

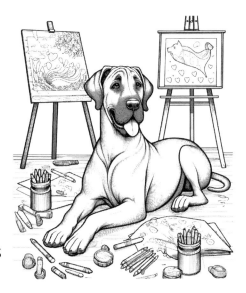

Plus, you'll get a complimentary copy of the "Don't Snooze Your Dreams" Audiobook as soon as it's released!

Scan the QR Code below or visiting

www.michelleweger.com/vip

Made in the USA
Columbia, SC
25 April 2025

43d938b5-33a4-44a0-b53d-afa341522734R01